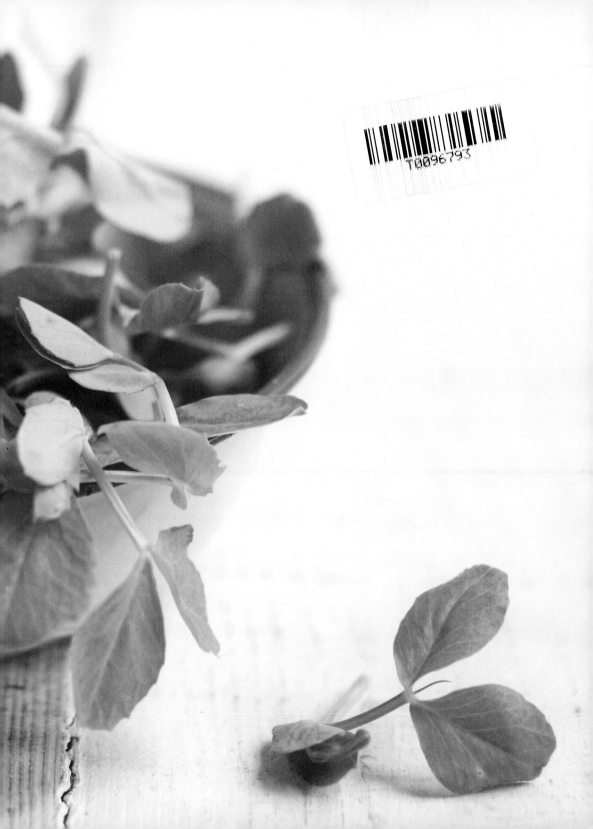

T0096793

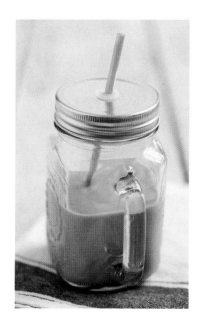

The Green Juice Book

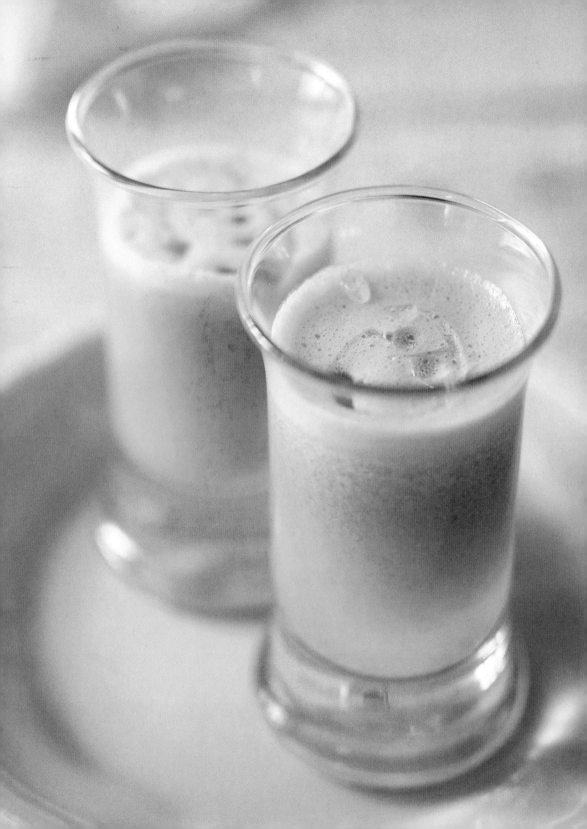

DETOX • ENERGIZE • LOSE WEIGHT

The Green Juice Book

Over 50 nutrition-packed all-green blends, with every recipe photographed

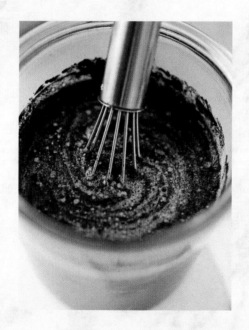

SARA LEWIS

PHOTOGRAPHY BY WILLIAM SHAW

LORENZ BOOKS

This edition is published by Lorenz Books,
an imprint of Anness Publishing Ltd,
108 Great Russell Street, London WC1B 3NA;
info@anness.com

www.lorenzbooks.com; www.annesspublishing.com;
twitter: @Anness_Books

If you like the images in this book and would
like to investigate using them for publishing,
promotions or advertising, please visit our website
www.practicalpictures.com for more information.

© Anness Publishing Ltd 2016

A CIP catalogue record for this book is available from
the British Library.

PUBLISHER: Joanna Lorenz
DESIGNER: Adelle Mahoney
PHOTOGRAPHY: William Shaw
FOOD FOR PHOTOGRAPHY: Sara Lewis
STYLING: Pene Parker
EDITORIAL: Sarah Lumby
PRODUCTION CONTROLLER: Pirong Wang

COOK'S NOTES
For all recipes, quantities are given in metric, imperial
measures and where appropriate, measures are also
given in standard cups and spoons. Follow one set, but
not a mixture because they are not interchangeable.
Standard spoon and cup measures are level.
1 tsp = 5ml, 1 tbsp = 15ml, 1 cup = 250ml/8fl oz.
Australian standard tablespoons are 20ml.
Australian readers should use 3 tsp in place of
1 tbsp for measuring small quantities.
American pints are 16fl oz/2 cups.
American readers should use 20fl oz/2.5 cups
in place of 1 pint when measuring liquids.
Garnishes and decorations are all optional and not
included in the nutritional analysis.

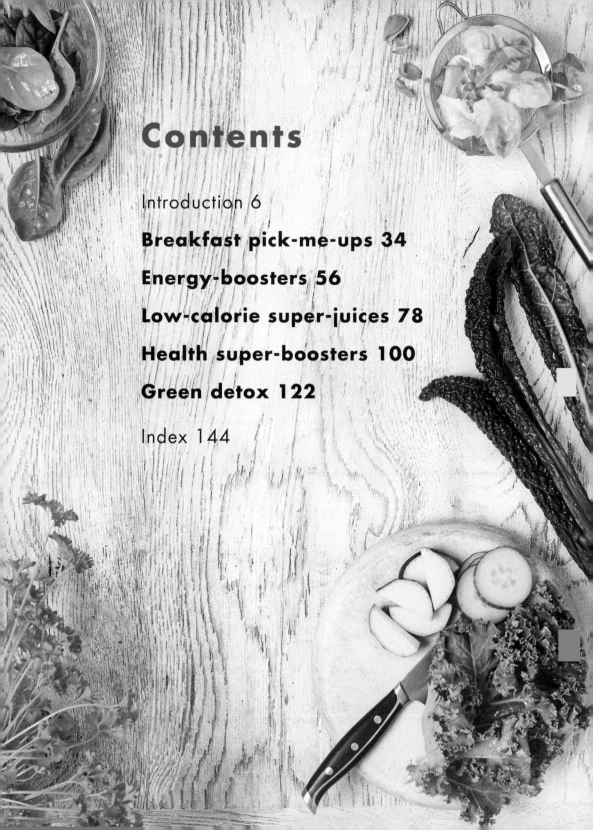

Contents

Introduction 6

Breakfast pick-me-ups 34

Energy-boosters 56

Low-calorie super-juices 78

Health super-boosters 100

Green detox 122

Index 144

10 minutes to change your life!

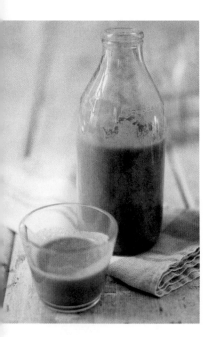

That's all it takes to make a healthy juice or shake-style drink, yet this very small and simple step can have a massive impact on your health and well-being.

When your body feels good you feel good; if you eat a diet of junk food, processed carbs and fizzy drinks you will feel sluggish, your skin will lose its vitality and if you are not already piling on the pounds and inches around your waistline, you very soon will be. With levels of obesity, type 2 diabetes, heart disease and cancer rising, it really is time to look at what you eat.

How often do you skip breakfast because you don't have time, or refuel at your desk on a hurried sandwich. Do you sit at the table with your family in the evening and enjoy the food you eat, or munch on the sofa in front of the television because you are too tired to talk?

We can all say we are too tired, too stressed, too busy to shop and buy healthy options – now is the time to stop making excuses and start making changes, and if you have picked up this book you are already thinking about doing it.

Introducing one healthy juice or shake a day is an easy way to boost nutrition levels to make you look and feel good, not just in the short term but as an easily maintained long-term lifestyle choice. We should all be eating at least five portions of vegetables and fruit a day but how many of us actually do? The reality is we should really be aiming for seven to eight. Australia recommends five portions of vegetables and two of fruit a day. Starting the day with a healthy juice or shake is a great way to boost vegetable and fruit intakes and these two food groups are at the core of the healthiest diets.

Enjoy foods as nature intended, avoiding refined processed foods, artificial chemical sweeteners, flavourings and preservatives. Replace with foods grown locally in a sustainable and environmentally friendly way. Aim to include foods from the main food groups of protein, good fats, complex carbs, vitamins and minerals, for optimum good health.

Try to be as healthy as you can – you don't have to ban cake or biscuits altogether, just to eat them in moderation, and keep as a

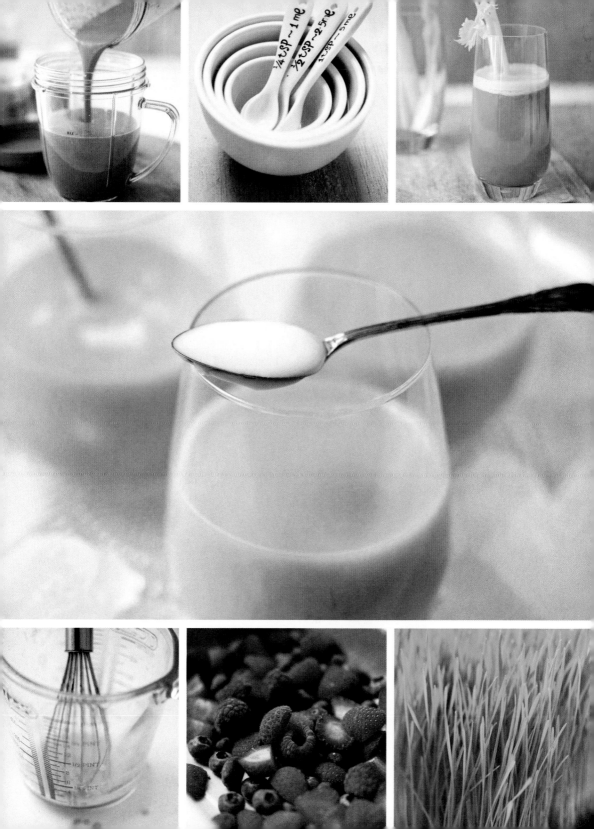

treat rather than everyday. Be aware of the sugar levels, and the healthy or non-healthy fats. You will have the odd bad day, but think of the week as a whole and once you embrace a healthier way of eating you will naturally find that you crave chips, cake and chocolate less.

What we eat does need to be taken into account with other factors such as age, build, lifestyle and activity levels. The old adage of a little of what you fancy does you good still rings true, it's just that we don't tend to eat little bits anymore. The key to maintaining a healthy diet is to enjoy your food and to eat a wide range of foods in moderation. Yes to juices but not in place of all meals: use a juice as one meal a day or as a healthy snack, perhaps drinking up to two juices a day to boost weight loss or aid a detox diet for a few days after an indulgent Christmas or holiday getaway.

The juices and smoothies in this book are packed with superfood nutrient-dense green vegetables, fruit, nuts and seeds. They are

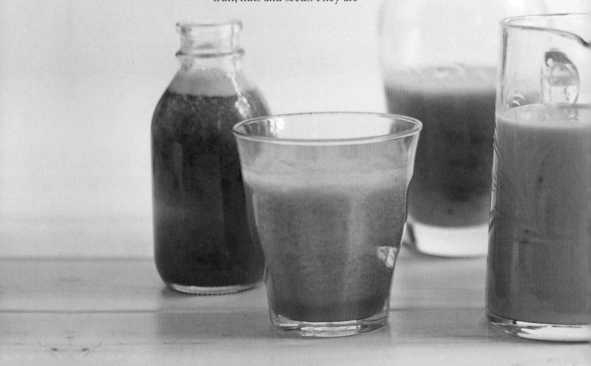

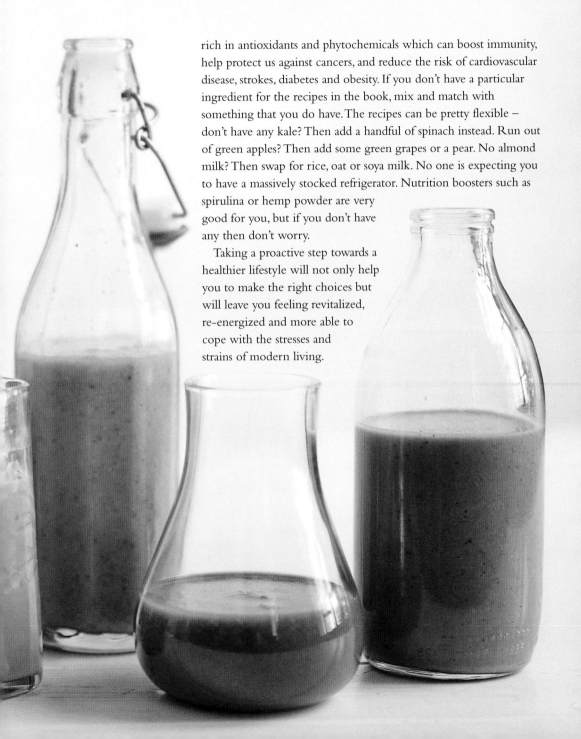

rich in antioxidants and phytochemicals which can boost immunity, help protect us against cancers, and reduce the risk of cardiovascular disease, strokes, diabetes and obesity. If you don't have a particular ingredient for the recipes in the book, mix and match with something that you do have. The recipes can be pretty flexible – don't have any kale? Then add a handful of spinach instead. Run out of green apples? Then add some green grapes or a pear. No almond milk? Then swap for rice, oat or soya milk. No one is expecting you to have a massively stocked refrigerator. Nutrition boosters such as spirulina or hemp powder are very good for you, but if you don't have any then don't worry.

Taking a proactive step towards a healthier lifestyle will not only help you to make the right choices but will leave you feeling revitalized, re-energized and more able to cope with the stresses and strains of modern living.

Why are green juices so good for us?

While we all know we should eat more healthily, few of us do, with most people barely eating 10% of our recommended dark green vegetables a day.

1 Juicing and smoothie-making is a great way to start new eating habits and start the ball rolling – for those who say they hate anything green, strong flavours can be disguised with clever blends of avocado, kiwi fruit, apple or pear.

2 The fear or hatred of green vegetables can be a psychological thing – maybe you remember being made to eat soggy cabbage for school lunches, suppers with overcooked green veggies that still haunt you, or perhaps overcooked Brussels sprouts on a Christmas menu. Changing the texture by juicing can create wonderful silky smooth blends that bear no resemblance to the original vegetable, surprising even the most sceptical. Spinach blends to a velvety smoothness and when mixed with avocado, banana or kiwi, is disguised in flavour, if not colour.

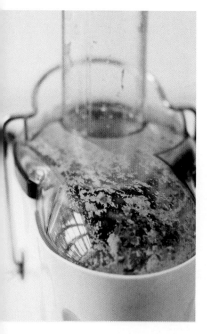
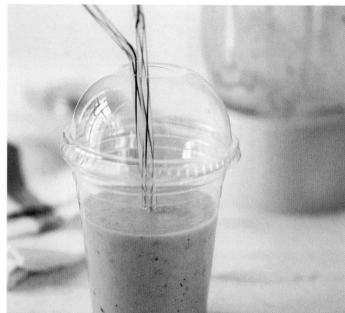

3 Processed foods, canned fizzy drinks (especially cola), coffee, red meat and some dairy foods can be very acidic – this is one of the reasons that the raw food diet has become such a hit. This diet promotes alkalinity and its devotees believe it aids digestion, boosts energy, and improves skin and mood. But in truth all food is acidic in the stomach and alkaline in the intestine, while urine pH levels will vary. What we eat will not affect the pH of our blood. Although there is little scientific evidence to back up the claims of the alkaline diet, those vegetables that feature highly in it, such as kale, spinach, watercress and cauliflower, and fruits such as apple, pear, mango, papaya, avocado and nuts, are nutrient-dense and adding them to a green juice is a great way to make our diet healthier.

4 As the vegetables have been juiced or blitzed in a blender, the drinks are easy to digest and their nutrients readily absorbed into the bloodstream. Vegetable-based juices and smoothies are a quick and easy way for busy people on the go to boost their health and well-being.

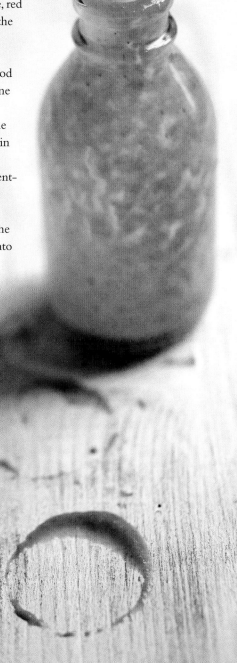

FIVE-A-DAY

There are two main ways to make a healthy green drink, by pressing a mix of vegetables and fruit through an electric juicer or by blending in a traditional liquidizer or a modern nutribullet-style individual smoothier-maker.

If you are making juice using an electric juicer one small 150ml/¼ pint/⅔ cup glass of unsweetened fruit or vegetable juice counts as one of your five-a-day. But one large glass doesn't count as two portions, as the fibre has been removed when pressed through the electric juicer.

A smoothie or shake-style drink may count as two, even three of your five-a-day as none of the fibre has been removed. 80g/3¼oz of fresh or frozen vegetables or fruit is counted as one of your five-a-day, but two portions of the same ingredient still only counts as one.

What makes up a healthy body

We need foods from each of the main food groups to keep our body in tip-top shape, and drinking a healthy smoothie, shake or juice is an easy way to do this.

POWER-PACKED PROTEINS

Protein is essential for our body, for growth, repair and maintenance of cells from everything from muscles and bones to hair and fingernails. It helps create enzymes that aid digestion, and produces antibodies that fight off infection and hormones that keep our body working properly. Proteins are broken down by the body during digestion into amino acids: there are 20 in total but only 8 can be obtained from the food we eat; the rest can be made by the body. Proteins cannot be stored in the body. If you don't have enough fats or carbs in your diet, your body proteins will be broken down and used as energy. Boost protein levels in your juices and shakes by adding nuts, pea protein powder, hemp powder or oil, soya milk, yogurt or tofu.

HURRAH FOR HEMP

Hemp makes a great addition to any juice or smoothie as it is one of the few plants that contains all 20 amino acids. Use in powdered form or as a cold pressed oil and stir in a little to a fresh juice or add to a shake before blending. Plus, it is rich in essential fatty acids omega 6 and 3 and a good source of vitamin E.

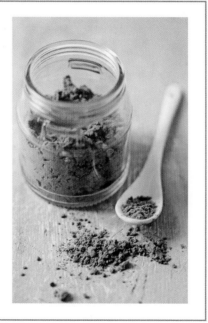

GOOD CARBS

Carbohydrates often get a bad press. We need carbs for energy rather like a car needs fuel to run, but just like fuel there are different grades. Refined white sugars and flours are often called empty carbs; they give the body a quick energy boost followed by a low-energy dip and very often leave us feeling sluggish. Usually found in cakes and pastries that are generally high in fats with little other nutrient benefit, it is these kind of carbs that give this food group a bad name.

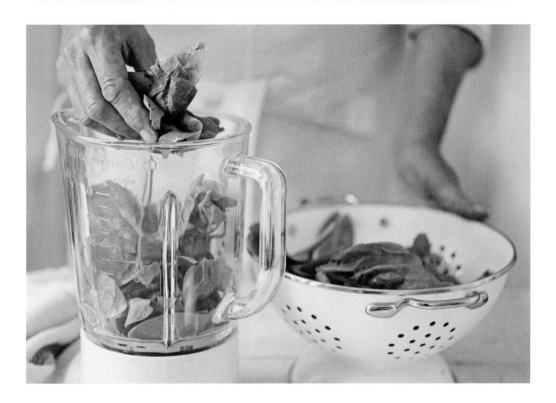

Complex carbs are the good guys, they take longer for the body to digest and include wholegrain flours, cereals, oats, barley, seeds, vegetables and fruit. As they take longer to digest these foods not only leave us feeling fuller for longer but they also give out a slowly released energy boost that helps to maintain blood sugar levels, to aid concentration and reduce fatigue. Unlike refined foods they are also rich in vitamins and minerals, while the high levels of fibre they contain help to maintain a healthy digestive system and help to reduce cholesterol.

ARE YOU SWEET ENOUGH?

Most of us have become very used to sweet things and when you first begin to juice and blend healthy vegetable shakes you may feel the need to add a little extra sweetness. Fruits vary in their natural sweetness, so if a juice tastes a little sharp you may prefer to substitute one of the ingredients with one that is a little sweeter next time, perhaps adding a kiwi fruit instead of celery or fennel. For drinks that have strong-tasting cabbage, spring greens or kale, you may like to drizzle in ½–1 tsp of clear honey, maple syrup or agave syrup into the drink at the end. If making a juice be mindful that those following a vegan diet will not add honey, so check first.

OATYLICIOUS

Just 1 tbsp of uncooked wholegrain rolled oats added to a shake-style smoothie equals one of the three daily recommended portions of wholegrains. 95% of people don't eat enough wholegrains and rather staggeringly one in three eat none at all. The risk of heart disease, stroke and type 2 diabetes may be up to 30% lower in people who regularly eat wholegrains as part of a low-fat healthy lifestyle.

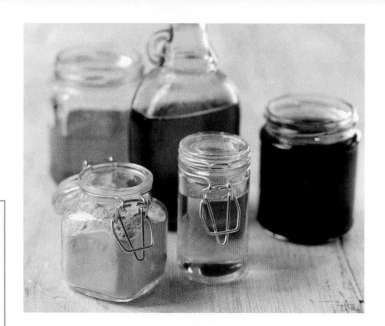

Clockwise from top left: Clear honey, maple, date and agave syrups and lacuma powder.

HAVE YOU TRIED LACUMA?

This fine beige-coloured powder is sold in health food stores and is made from the Peruvian lacuma fruit. When dried and ground it has a maple syrup-like flavour that is low on the glycaemic index and also contains a range of vitamins, minerals and fibre.

You might also like to try date syrup, sometimes called date honey, a rich thick syrup popular in the Middle East and made from pressed dates, agave syrup, natural honey or maple syrup. Check the label before buying budget-priced maple syrup as the bottles are not always pure maple syrup but mixed with high-fructose corn syrup. As with any sweetener, use sparingly.

You might also like to try adding a little powdered palm or coconut sugar. Powdered sugar substitutes, the kind you add to tea or coffee, can be strong-tasting and overwhelm the natural flavours of a healthy juice or shake and somehow don't sit with the wholefood ethos of natural juices and shakes.

As your palate begins to adjust to this new healthy way of eating and drinking you will naturally find that you no longer crave such sweet things. It is feared by some health professionals that high levels of sugar in our diet may become as great a problem as alcohol consumption. Our generation consumes three times the amount of fructose than 50 years ago.

Being aware of the amounts of sugar that you consume in foods is key, only then can you start to reduce the amounts of sugar in your diet. The average adult should have around 260g/9¼oz of carbohydrates a day, of which a maximum 90g/3½oz is from sugars. Ideally we should be aiming to reduce this down to 7 teaspoons a day from the foods that we eat.

It is better to make small positive changes and gradually try to reduce sugar levels week on week rather than to try and do it overnight and fail miserably.

HEALTHY FATS

Weight for weight fats contain more than twice the amount of calories as carbohydrates or protein. Yet we need fat as a necessary part of every cell to help absorb fat-soluble vitamins A, D, E and K, to provide essential fatty acids and as a concentrated form of energy. The important thing is to get the right kind of fats and in the right proportion. Adding half an avocado or a small drizzle of cold-pressed avocado oil, hemp or almond oil can be a great way to boost energy levels in smoothies and juices with mono- or polyunsaturated fats rather than saturated ones.

VITAMINS

Vegetables and fruit are rich in these complex substances vital for good health, and as many chemical reactions cannot take place in the body without them, they are vital catalysts. B vitamins are needed for the release of energy and for healthy nerve and muscle function. Beta-carotene, vitamin C and vitamin E are also antioxidants and they act like our natural bodyguard to help fight free-radical damage and to help protect against cancer and heart disease, as well as to reduce the risk of age-related diseases such as cataracts, Alzheimer's and Parkinson's disease.

MINERALS

The minerals zinc, selenium, copper and manganese also make up the team of antioxidants that help prevent free-radical damage. Minerals help regulate bodily fluids, make up enzymes and are involved in metabolic processes. Just a handful of dark green leafy vegetables or a tablespoon of dried sea vegetables is all it takes to boost our daily multi-mineral intake, while avocados add a manganese boost, bananas add potassium and nuts add selenium.

COCONUT OIL, GOOD OR BAD?

Coconut fat has been gaining in popularity as the must-have health food, but beware, as it is loaded with saturated fat which we are advised to reduce and replace with unsaturated fats as an effective way of reducing blood cholesterol. Much better to choose coconut water or low-fat coconut milk when making healthy smoothies and shakes.

DRINK IN A RAINBOW

The brighter the colour of the vegetable or fruit, the more cancer-protecting antioxidants there are.

Below, clockwise from top: Chia, sesame, sunflower, pumpkin and ground flaxseeds. Below right: Goji berries.

SEEDS AND SUPER NUTRIENTS

Sunflower, sesame and pumpkin seeds – these help boost protein, B vitamins, vitamin E and fibre. They are quite high in calories at 100 per tablespoon but add an energy- and nutrient-dense addition to any drink.

Flaxseeds – sometimes called linseeds, these contain omega 3 and 6 essential fatty acids, plus magnesium, manganese, vitamin B and fibre. They are one of the best food sources of lignans, which are rich in antioxidants and act as phytoestrogens which help to balance hormone levels.

Chia seeds – these little black wonder seeds add protein, fibre, omega 3 fatty acids, plus calcium, iron, copper and zinc. When mixed with liquid they form a gel, so drink as soon as you have made the juice or shake.

Spirulina – this dark blue-green powder is made from dried algae and contains 60% protein, vitamin B12, a difficult vitamin to get for those on a vegan diet, plus essential fatty acids. It is also thought to have immune-boosting properties and may help to normalize blood pressure. Chlorella, also an algae, is similar to spirulina but has a hard cell wall that needs to be broken down during manufacture so that the body can absorb it during digestion.

Green tea – this is thought to contain more antioxidant polyphenols than black tea. Matcha green tea is sold in a concentrated powdered form and contains 137 times the amount of antioxidants of regular green tea.

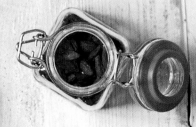

Wheatgrass – a little goes a long way so buy in powdered form for convenience or fresh-grown in seed trays from good health food stores or organic farm shops. It contains all 8 essential amino acids plus B vitamins, vitamin C, E and K and iron.

Baobab superfruit – rich in potassium, calcium, vitamin C, antioxidants and iron, this coconut-sized fruit is sold in a dried and powdered form and is thought to also aid digestion and enhance the growth of probiotic bacteria in the gut.

Goji berries – these tiny bright red dried fruits are rich in carotenes which help to boost our immune system and may even help protect against heart disease and cancer.

CACAO VS. COCOA?

Raw cacao is made by cold pressing unroasted cocoa beans, so removing the fat and retaining important antioxidants, minerals and the amino acid tryptophan which aids relaxation and sleep. Cocoa powder looks the same but it has been roasted at high temperatures, so lowering the overall nutritional value and giving it a stronger and slightly bitter flavour.

Above, clockwise from top: Wheatgrass powder, matcha green tea, baobab powder, spirulina.

STAYING HYDRATED

Drinking water is key to staying healthy. At birth the human body is 70% water and this decreases with age. Women should aim for at least 1.6 litres/2½ pints, men 2 litres/3½ pints of water a day to help prevent constipation, kidney stones and urinary tract infections. If you don't drink enough you will become tired, have poor concentration, headaches and may feel dizzy and light-headed. While water is the top of the list, fresh juices and shakes add an important vitamin- and mineral-boosting contribution; just be aware of the amounts of natural sugar they contain so drink no more than two juices a day plus glasses of tap, filtered or bottled water. Herb teas, tea and coffee also count.

Age, gender, build, lifestyle and activity not to mention the weather also affect how much we need to drink, so too do warm and dry environments such as air-conditioned offices or centrally-heated homes.

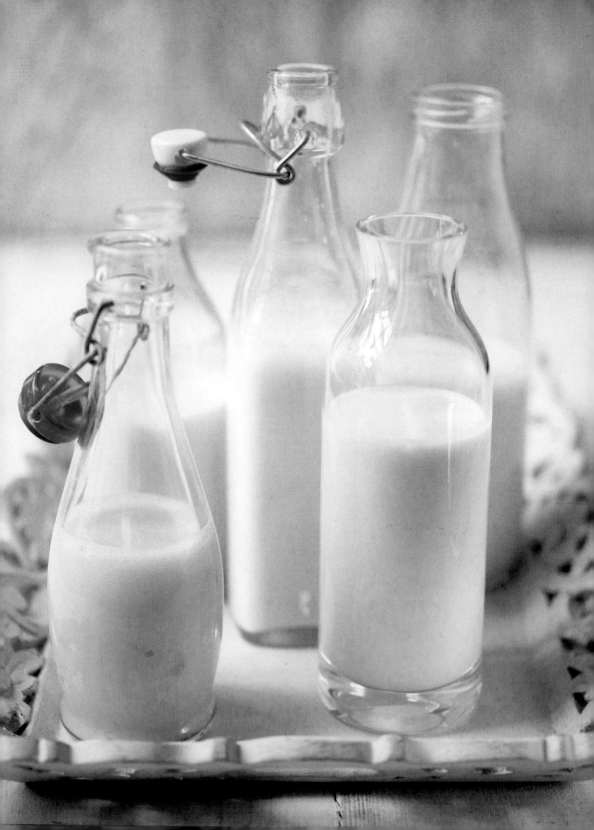

DAIRY-FREE MILKS

Dairy-free milks have been growing in popularity and are no longer the milk of choice only for those who are allergic to dairy or following a vegan diet. These lactose-free milks are now widely available in all supermarkets in longlife or fresh cartons, sweetened or unsweetened. For juices and shakes choose the unsweetened versions and add natural sweetness with fruits and vegetables. They are all fortified with added calcium, some also have vitamin B12 (a vitamin difficult to obtain on a vegetarian diet), vitamin B2 and vitamin D.

MAKING YOUR OWN NUT MILKS

Although readily available in supermarkets you might also like to try making your own nut milks at home.

Add 125g/4½oz/1 cup unblanched almonds (with brown skins), roughly chopped, or the same weight of cashew nut pieces, to a large plastic container and cover with 1 litre/1¾ pints/4 cups cold filtered water. Cover and leave to soak overnight.

Transfer to a blender, in batches if needed, and blitz until smooth. Strain through a sieve or strainer lined with muslin or cheesecloth. You should have 1 litre/1¾ pints/4 cups of nut milk. Pour the strained liquid into a bottle, seal and keep in the refrigerator up to 2 days. If it separates, simply stir before use.

The remaining nut meal can be kept and a tablespoon or two added to shakes or smoothie-style drinks, and stirred into breakfast muesli, granola, porridge or vegetable curries.

MAKING SUBSTITUTIONS

While the recipes in this book list specific vegetables, fruit, nuts, seeds and liquid – either water or unsweetened almond milk – think of this as a starting point. If you don't have a particular ingredient, swap for something that you do have. If you don't have any coconut water, then just use ordinary water. Unsweetened almond milk

Opposite, from left to right: Oat, soya (behind oat), hemp, almond and rice milks.

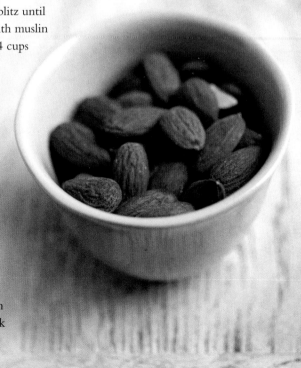

can be interchanged with oat or rice milk, just make sure to choose unsweetened varieties. Soya milk has a slightly stronger flavour, so this is down to personal choice.

Dairy yogurts have been chosen for the best flavour, but do by all means swap for dairy-free versions. Almonds, cashew nuts and hazelnuts are all interchangeable. Brazil nuts may also be used but have a much stronger flavour, again down to personal taste. Seeds such as pumpkin, sesame, sunflower and linseeds are all interchangeable. The key here is to make sure they are finely ground, either in the blender along with the other ingredients or grind small quantities of the ones that you use the most and keep in a small covered container in the refrigerator. Packs of ready-ground flaxseeds or mixed seeds are available in supermarkets but it is much cheaper to grind your own at home either in a liquidizer or spice mill.

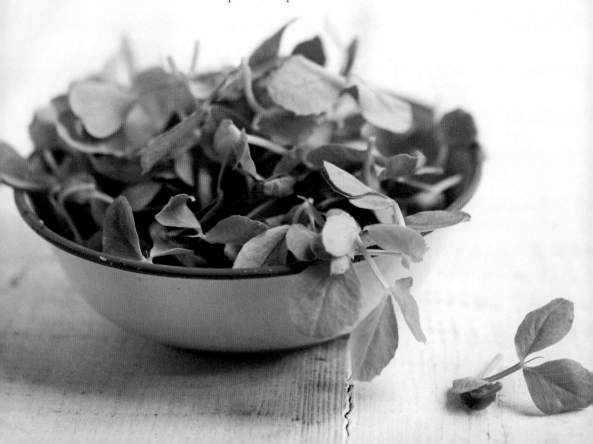

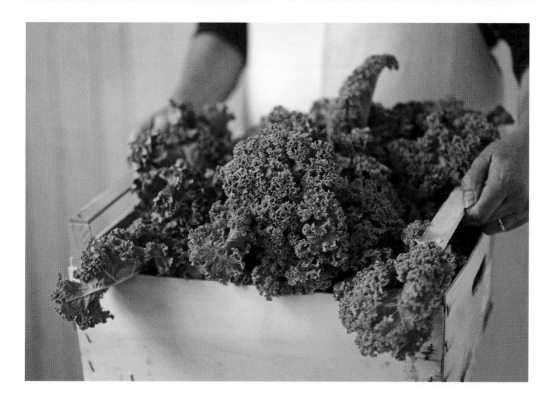

GOING ORGANIC

Once you embrace the healthy eating ethos, buying organic vegetables and fruit is the next natural step. Buying organic meat is a huge financial jump from the ordinary supermarket alternatives but choosing organically grown vegetables, fruit, nuts, seeds and yogurt is not much more expensive.

'Organic farmers take a more holistic, principled approach that respects processes to build positive health across the ecology of the farm', says the Soil Association. Pesticides are severely restricted and GM foods banned. Rather than using artificial oil-based fertilizers, farmers rotate crops and enrich the soil with compost, manure and clover.

If you have a garden, why not grow your own. It is a great way to encourage the whole family to think about the food that they eat, and an easy and cheap way to eat organic produce. Popping out to the garden to pick some ultra-fresh salad leaves, a cabbage or some broccoli means that vitamins and minerals are at their highest levels. In the "Dig for Victory" and "Victory Gardens" campaigns of World War II, the UK and US governments encouraged families to cultivate their own kale as it was such a prolific, hardy and almost idiot-proof vegetable for first-time gardeners to grow.

Above: The best way to ensure your kale is organic is to buy from your local farm shop or have a go at growing your own.

Making smoothies

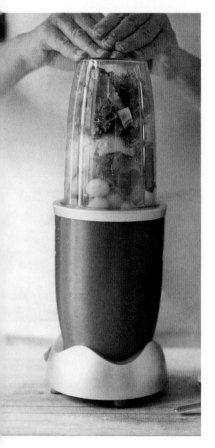

For those who prefer thick shake or smoothie-style drinks a good blender is the way to go, and has the benefits of the retained fibre.

Whereas juicers extract the nutritional essence from your vegetables and fruits they leave behind a small amount of dense pulp; in a blender this is retained, which means a thicker textured drink that includes the natural benefits of the fibre. For smoothie drinks everything that is added to the blender goblet is kept in the drink, making this a truly high-fibre option with very little waste.

Blenders vary greatly in motor power and speed, settings, jug or pitcher size, and price. A Vitamix is the super de-luxe machine, although it comes with a pretty hefty price tag. It will blitz even the most robust of veggies and rock-hard ice cubes to an ultra-smooth drink in seconds, plus it is great for making instant dairy-free ice cream with frozen bananas, soups, and superfine ground seed and nut mixes. But unless you cook a lot, or want to make drinks for more than one person, you may prefer a smaller nutribullet-style blender. These come with two different-sized goblets plus screw-on lids so that you can take the smoothie to work or to the gym after blending. They also have an additional blade for grinding nuts and seeds.

Whatever machine you choose make sure that it is easy to put together and take apart, that it can go in the dishwasher and that you have counter-space in the kitchen to leave it out. If you store the machine in the cupboard, chances are you won't use it on a daily basis.

BLENDER TIPS
- Avocados, bananas, papaya, mangoes, summer berries and blueberries are best blitzed in a blender or nutribullet rather than an electric juicer.
- Always add liquid – either water, non-dairy milks or yogurt.
- If your blender isn't very powerful, grind nuts and seeds separately then mix into the remaining ingredients.
- Don't overfill the blender goblet and always fix the lid on firmly before use.

1 Prepare and add your green ingredients to the blender goblet.
2 Pour in liquid – water, coconut water, non-dairy milks or yogurt.
3 Screw on the blender lid then blitz until smooth.
4 Pour into a glass and serve.

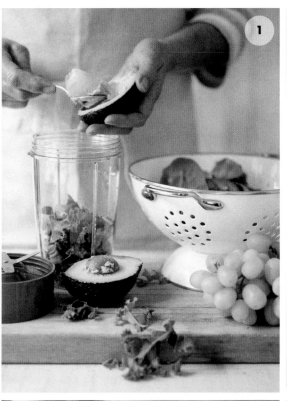

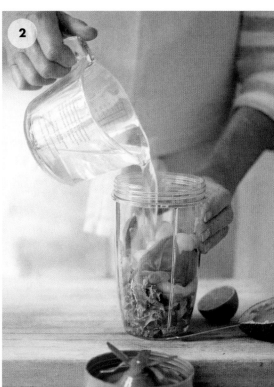

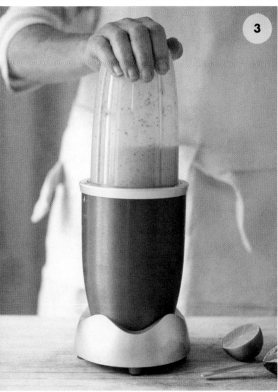

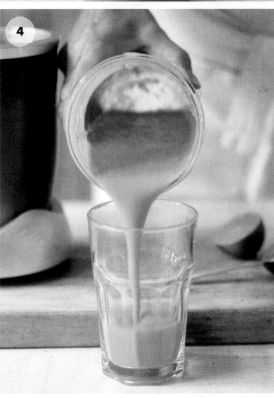

Making juices

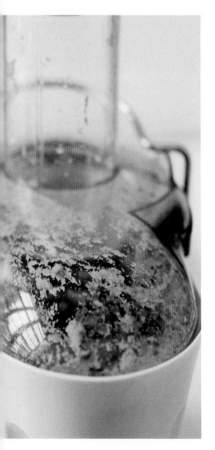

Juices are made by pressing vegetables and fruit through an electric juicer; as most of the fibre is removed they rarely need any additional liquid to be added.

An electric juicer looks a little like a food processor and you really do get what you pay for. These machines generally come with a clear top with a chute to feed vegetables and fruit through to a wire basket with teeth, which spins to extract the juice into a separate jug or pitcher, and with the fruit pith, peel and seeds going into a separate container. Choose a machine with a wide chute so that apples and pears don't need to be cut into pieces, and ideally with two speeds – low for extracting as much juice as possible from soft fleshy leaves and a higher speed setting for harder vegetables such as carrots, beetroot or parsnips.

If you plan to extract the juice from fresh wheatgrass then a masticating juicer is worth considering. This looks like a mincing or grinding machine and crushes the vegetables with a rotating screw to extract the juice. They are quite slow to use and expensive.

For fans of fresh orange juice, an electric citrus press may be for you. Some larger food processors come with this as a standard attachment and they make light work of squeezing the juice from oranges, lemons and limes. Rather than buying a separate machine, trim away the zest and pith from citrus fruit and either press the fruit through an electric juicer or roughly chop the fruit to add to a blender or nutribullet.

1 Add ingredients to the juicer feeder chute.

2 Extract the juice.

3 Separate the machine.

JUICER TIPS

- Trim off the zest and most of the pith before adding citrus fruits to a juicer or blender or the juice will taste bitter.
- Peel kiwi fruit and pineapple before juicing.
- Add kale, spinach or herbs to the juicer chute first then add the other vegetables and fruit to extract as much juice out of them as possible.
- If you don't have time to wash the juicer parts before going out, put into a bowl of water to soak.

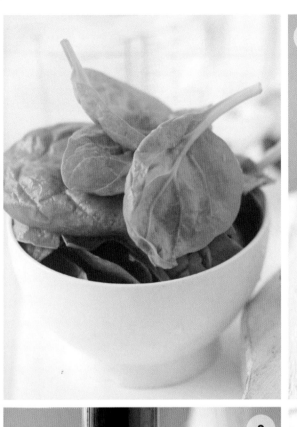

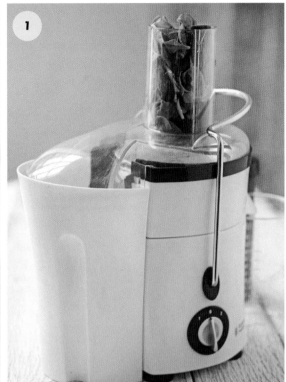

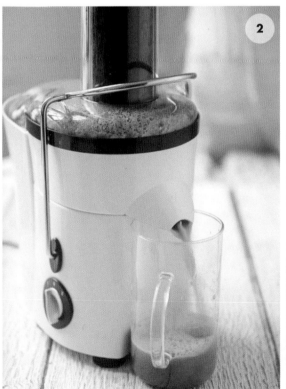

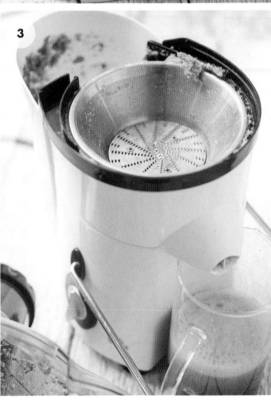

A–Z of core green ingredients

The best-tasting juices and smoothies are made with a mix of green vegetables and green fruits, the natural sweetness of the fruit helping to balance the stronger flavours of kale, cabbage or celery. But it doesn't mean that non-green ingredients are off the list. Far from it, just bear in mind that beetroot, carrots, strawberries or blueberries taste great but tend to muddy the colours, giving more of a khaki or army-issue shade of green.

Avocados – Thought to be one of the most nutritionally complete fruits, avocados are rich in concentrated energy in the form of monounsaturated fats, plus vitamin B6 needed to aid energy release. They have more potassium than bananas, to help regulate blood pressure and lower the risk of heart attacks and strokes, and are rich in vitamin E with smaller amounts of vitamin C and lutein, all powerful antioxidants. Avocados add a wonderful velvety creaminess to smoothie-style drinks, or you can drizzle a little avocado oil into a drink made in a juicer.

Apples – Choose green-skinned apples for natural energy-boosting sweetness. The pectin they contain helps to lower cholesterol and helps to activate beneficial bacteria in the large intestine, while adding vitamin C too. When added to blender-style drinks they also boost fibre levels.

Broccoli – The darker the florets, irrespective of them being green, deep blue-green or purple, the higher the amounts of vitamin C and beta-carotene which the body converts into vitamin A. Broccoli also contains beneficial indoles – nitrogen compounds which may help to protect DNA from damage and so protect against cancer. Don't throw the stems away when juicing; although you won't get masses of juice, what you will get will be super-concentrated.

Citrus fruits – Choose from limes, lemons, grapefruit and oranges for a fresh tangy flavour and vitamin C boost to help

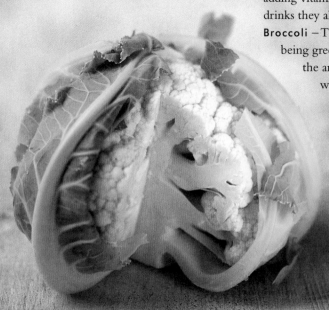

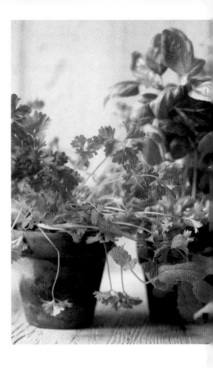

fight infection, aid healing and promote healthy teeth, gums, skin, bones and cartilage. Vitamin C cannot be stored by the body so is needed on a daily basis.

Cabbages – These are rich in vitamin C for boosting immunity, vitamin K for strong bones and healthy blood clotting, the folates required for cell division and formation of DNA, plus vitamin E to help reduce free-radical damage and potassium to help regulate blood pressure. The flavour is quite strong so a little goes a long way when juicing. Spring greens/collards are also part of the cabbage family.

Cauliflowers – Like broccoli, cauliflower belongs to the cruciferous family and provides good sources of sulphurous compounds which may help protect against cancer. Also try Romanesco, a green cauliflower that has similar nutritional values.

Celery – These stems were first used by Roman physicians as a gentle and effective diuretic and as a treatment for kidney and urinary infections. Celery also contains an anti-inflammatory so may help relieve the symptoms of gout. Don't trim off the leaves but add these to smoothies and juices too. Although high in water and very low in calories, celery has a surprisingly strong flavour so add just one stem to a drink.

Courgettes/zucchini – High in water to aid hydration, courgettes add a mild flavour that balances stronger-flavoured fruit and vegetables when juiced.

Cucumbers – Although made up of a staggering 95% water, cucumber is low in calories and aids hydration when added to juices. It also acts as a mild diuretic. Green-fleshed melons also aid hydration.

Green grapes – Fresh, tangy and good in either a juicer or blender, a handful of grapes or 100g/3¾oz contains just 60 calories, so makes a good low-calorie addition to any drink, as well as being a good source of potassium to help regulate blood pressure.

Herbs – Choose from parsley, coriander/cilantro, mint and basil for a chlorophyll-boosting, detoxing addition to juices or smoothies. Parsley contains useful amounts of vitamin C and iron and can help as a breath freshener while mint aids digestion. Coriander leaves also aid digestion and add a spicy tang to juices. Basil acts as a natural tranquilizer and is thought by herbalists to calm the nervous system, aid digestion and ease stomach cramps.

Above: Herbs shouldn't be missed out of green juices; have a selection to-hand growing in pots in your kitchen.

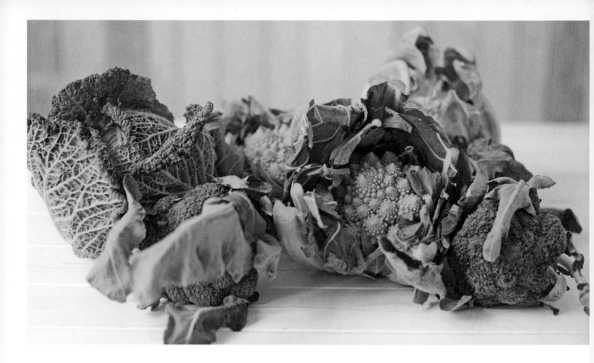

Above: Cabbage, Romanesco
cauliflower, cauliflower and broccoli.

Kale – This robust hardy vegetable has grown in popularity over recent years. Sometimes called curly kale or Scotch kale, look out for red Russian kale with its frilly leaves and the Italian black kale known as cavolo nero. Easy to grow by even the novice gardener it is rich in lutein and zeaxanthin, two cancer-fighting antioxidants, plus vitamins C and K, chlorophyll and iron which helps with the oxygenation and health of blood cells so helping to fight fatigue. If you are new to adding kale to drinks, introduce slowly so that your body can get used to it and avoid the possibility of flatulence. Buy as whole leaves or bags of ready-shredded to save time.

Kiwi fruit – Packed with immune-boosting vitamin C and a good source of potassium, kiwis are also a good source of cancer-fighting antioxidants. This fruit is great in a juicer or blender.

Lettuce – Choose darker green leaves for the most nutritional value. As the leaves have such a high water content the calories are low. Amounts of vitamins C and K vary between types of lettuce, with romaine lettuce containing some of the highest levels. Also try Little Gem/Bibb, romaine, Webb's Wonder and lamb's lettuce/mâché.

Pears – The delicate sweetness of pears make a great addition in juices or smoothies to balance out stronger-tasting vegetables, while the natural pectin they contain can help to reduce cholesterol. No need to peel or core before use, choose just-ripe pears for the best flavour.

Pea shoots – Young pea shoots or baby peas still in their pods are naturally sweet and delicious in smoothies.

Rocket/arugula – Related to kale, rocket contains powerful antioxidants, an excellent source of vitamins C and K, plus folates, copper and iron. It contains much more flavour than lettuce leaves with a peppery taste a little like watercress.

Sea vegetables – the Japanese have been harvesting sea vegetables for centuries. They are rich in the iodine needed for normal functioning of the thyroid gland, and smaller amounts of copper and iron for healthy blood, magnesium for proper function of muscles and nerves, calcium for healthy bones, potassium for balance of fluids and zinc for the body's immune system. Look out for packs of mixed dried and shredded sea vegetables that include dried dulce, nori and sea lettuce or packs of shredded dulce. There is no need to soak them in liquid before use, simply add to the blender when making shake or smoothie-style drinks.

Spinach – Although we always think of spinach being a good source of iron, it is not as good as you might imagine. It does however contain a high concentration of carotenoids, including beta-carotene and lutein which may help protect against cancer. Plus it also contains potassium and folate. Baby spinach leaves are low in oxalates; as the leaves grow so the amount of oxalates increases and this can inhibit the absorption of calcium and iron from the leaves. Spinach adds a wonderful dark green to juices and blends to an ultra-smooth velvety texture in smoothies. Try also chard with deep green leaves and white or rainbow-coloured stems.

Watercress – These leaves are rich in vitamin K needed for bone-building and strengthening, and vitamin A for good eye health. It also contains the antioxidants lutein and zeaxanthin.

Wheatgrass – Buy as sprouted grass in trays or in powdered form; wheatgrass is rich in chlorophyll, protein and the vitamins A, C, E, K and B12, plus a range of minerals.

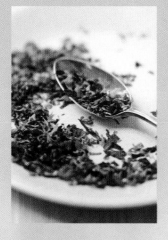

Above: Mixed dried and shredded sea vegetables can be found in packets on the shelves of good health or wholefood stores.

Kickstart your diet

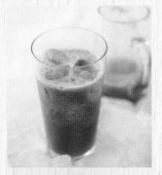

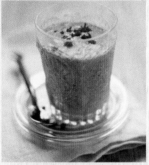

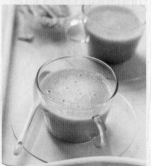

Drinking a juice or healthy shake can be a great way to kickstart a diet. Just one healthy juice or smoothie for breakfast and one for lunch followed by a light low-calorie stir-fry, salad or veggie-rich casserole can help you break bad eating habits and get you started on your diet. Then once the weight begins to come off, have just one healthy juice or shake a day.

DIET PLAN

If you have been on a diet for a while and your weight loss has plateaued then including one or two low-calorie shakes or juices can help super-power you to your goal. Once there, don't stop juicing: by including a healthy juice or shake once each day you will be able to maintain your new slim self and stay in optimum health.

STAY ON TRACK...

• Make a plan and a time scale that you think you can stick to.
• Shop cleverly and work out which juices and smoothies you plan to do along with healthy meal options. Go shopping with a list and never shop when you are hungry.
• Get rid of those snacks and bars of chocolate in the cupboard. If temptation isn't there you can't be tempted. If you do slip up, don't give up but try to get back on track.
• Drink plenty of water in addition to healthy juices and smoothies.
• Write down exactly what you eat in a day – just the action of adding to the list can make you think twice: am I really hungry, do I really want that, or can I wait a while.

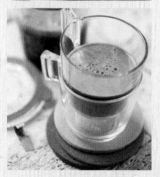

Left, top to bottom: Green Goddess, Hormone Balance, Citrus Burst, Citrus Beet Blast. Opposite: Cacao Comforter.

MONDAY
Breakfast Green Giant
Lunch Blueberry Booster
Supper Prawn/shrimp stir-fry with a bag of ready-prepared vegetables, a little spray-oil, soy sauce and chopped coriander/cilantro. Serve with rice.

TUESDAY
Breakfast Zingy Refresher
Lunch Healthy Heart
Supper Shepherd's pie made with turkey, ready-diced swede/rutabaga and carrot, stock and dried herbs then topped with potatoes mashed with skimmed milk and no butter. Top brushed with beaten egg and baked.

WEDNESDAY
Breakfast Swiss Mix
Lunch Green Goddess
Supper Grilled salmon with jumbo potato salad made with sliced just-cooked new potatoes tossed with chopped herbs, chopped spring onions/scallions, low-fat plain yogurt and rocket/arugula leaves with a side of halved cherry tomatoes drizzled with a little balsamic vinegar.

THURSDAY
Breakfast Good Morning Shake
Lunch Citrus Beet Blast
Supper Baked potato topped with skinny coleslaw made with plain yogurt and just 1 tsp mayonnaise per portion, grated carrot, diced apple, shredded red cabbage and a spoonful of corn, topped with a handful of salad leaves and flaked tuna canned in springwater.

FRIDAY
Breakfast Wake-up Call
Lunch Hormone Balance
Supper Couscous salad with diced tomatoes, chopped bell peppers, cucumber, chopped herbs and a lemon vinaigrette made with just 1 tbsp olive oil, spooned over salad and topped with 25g/1oz crumbled feta cheese per portion.

SATURDAY
Breakfast Citrus Burst
Lunch Green Tornado
Supper Garlicky grilled steak, with all the fat removed, blanched potato wedges sprinkled with Cajun spices and sprayed with oil then oven baked, and served with salad.

Or, turkey chilli with butternut squash and canned red kidney beans, served with brown rice, a spoonful of low-fat plain yogurt and a simple salsa with diced red onion, tomato and chopped coriander/cilantro leaves.

SUNDAY
Breakfast Cacao Comforter
Lunch Super-green Vitality
Supper Roast chicken eaten without the skin, baby new potatoes roasted with fresh rosemary and a little spray oil, served with flour-free gravy and a selection of baby carrots, asparagus and green beans.

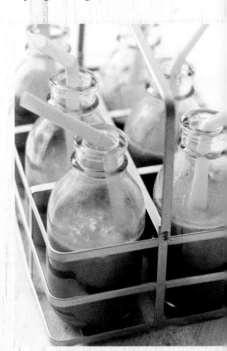

Detoxing with green juices

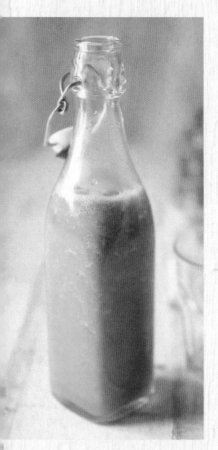

If you are feeling tired and sluggish then your body could be trying to tell you that it needs a break. Your body is a finely-tuned engine that needs the right kinds of foods to function at its optimum level. Cut out the junk and processed foods. Reduce the amount of tea and coffee, make the decision to cut out the cigarettes if you do smoke, exercise more and catch up on sleep.

To help your body rid itself of the build-up of processed foods it can be helpful to go on a detox diet, to cut out red meat, dairy foods, gluten-based flours and grains, and refined sugars, and increase the amount of water that you drink each day.

On the internet you will find many crash diets that advocate drinking nothing other than juices for three or five days and some even longer. This kind of extreme diet is not recommended by nutritionists and dietitians and comes with a myriad of unwelcome side effects ranging from headaches, dizziness, constipation or frequent dashes to the bathroom. It is much better to introduce one or two green juices or smoothies a day with a healthy main meal for lunch or supper. If you are new to juicing you may still experience 'juice breath' as you adjust to a diet rich in kale and spinach but by adding cucumber, parsley or mint to your drinks this can be greatly reduced.

Green juices are crammed with a huge range of flavours and tastes. Start the diet over a weekend to give your body time to relax and unwind and make yourself the number-one priority. Catch up on some boxed television series, or that film you have been meaning to watch but haven't had the time for. Enjoy a peaceful walk and some early nights. When we are stressed and tired it shows in our faces, but forget about the facelift and start making changes from the inside out.

As with all dietary lifestyle changes seek medical advice before replacing meals with juices or shakes if you are pregnant, suffer with kidney stones, have chronic illness or are on long-term medication, if you suffer with blood sugar imbalances or diabetes.

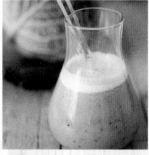

SATURDAY
Breakfast Totally Tropical
Lunch Red Cabbage and Kale
Digestive Aid
Supper Brown rice risotto
with pumpkin and sage

SUNDAY
Breakfast Green Giant
Lunch Gorgeous Green
Pep-up
Supper Laksa with rice
noodles and tofu

MONDAY
Breakfast Zingy Refresher
Lunch Stamina Maximizer
Supper Raw sprouted salad
with diced beet, grated
carrot, diced bell peppers,
nuts and quinoa in a lemon
juice dressing.

TUESDAY
Breakfast Parslied Purifier
Lunch Cacao and Avocado
Smoothie
Supper Lentil dahl with a side
dish of potatoes and spinach

WEDNESDAY
Breakfast Swiss Mix
Lunch Citrus Super Cleanse
Supper Tomato and squash
curry with brown rice

THURSDAY
Breakfast Good Morning
Shake
Lunch Creamy Apple and
Parsnip Soother
Supper Warm puy lentil
salad with balsamic vinegar
and chopped parsley, topped
with rosemary and garlic-
roasted bell peppers and
courgettes/zucchini

FRIDAY
Breakfast Wake-up Call
Lunch Summer Herb Sensation
Supper Vegetable chilli with
brown rice and roasted
butternut squash

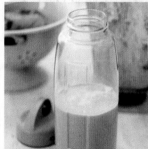

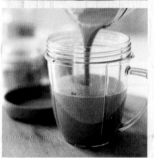

This detox plan replaces
two meals with a juice or
smoothie for a short detox.
For longer than five to
seven days, add a light
snack at breakfast or
lunchtime for a more
balanced diet.

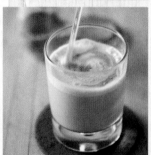

Right, top to bottom: Gorgeous Green
Pep-up, Stamina Maximizer, Cacao and
Avocado Smoothie, Creamy Apple
and Parsnip Soother, Summer
Herb Sensation. Opposite: Gingered
Pineapple Revitalizer.

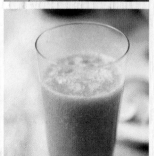

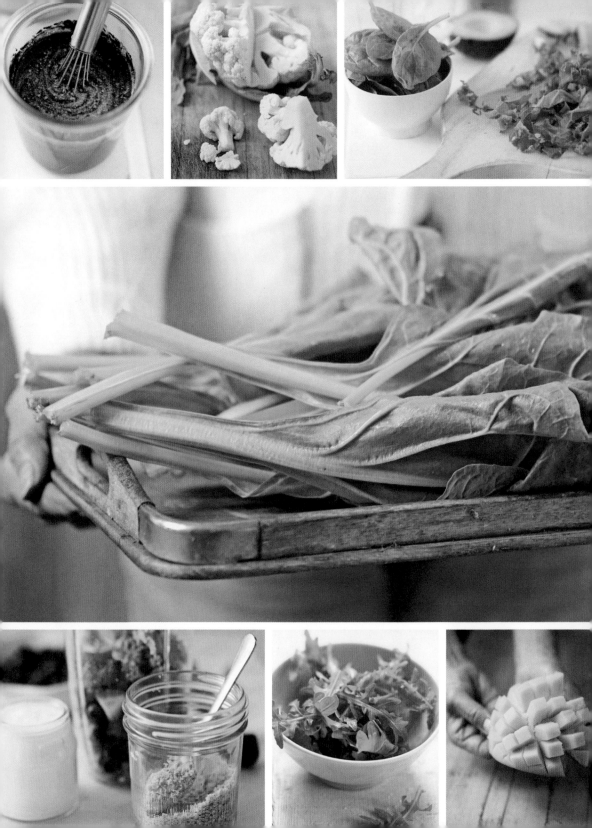

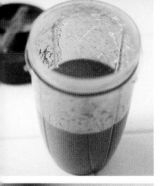

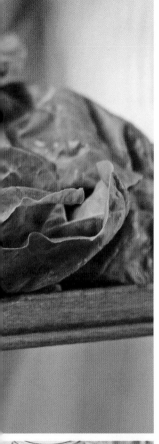

BREAKFAST PICK-ME-UPS

It's all too easy to get up late and skip breakfast, but this meal is vitally important to energize and refuel your body for the busy day ahead. Set your alarm clock 10 minutes earlier and make time to blitz a healthy juice or smoothie, it really doesn't take much longer to do than pouring milk over a sugary cereal and is much healthier for you. Once you begin to make your own juices you will feel and look so much better and if you really are short of time, then take the juice to work with you.

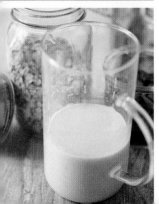

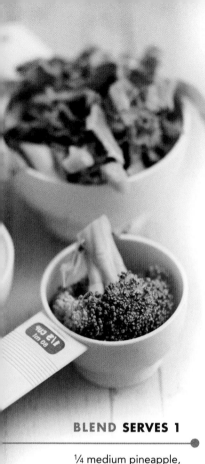

Totally tropical

A mild, soothing smoothie with just a hint of ginger, this healthy drink is packed with fibre and natural fruit sugars to kickstart the day and provide slow-release energy to help avoid mood swings and aid concentration at work.

1 Add all the fruit and vegetables to the blender goblet. Add the ginger then pour in the coconut milk and water. Add the lid and blitz until smooth.

2 If your blender goblet is small then add just half the water and blitz until smooth then adjust to the desired thickness with the remaining water.

3 Pour into a tall glass and serve.

COOK'S TIP – Ginger has long been thought to aid travel sickness but it can also help those suffering with morning sickness in pregnancy or recovering from illness.

NUTRIENT NOTE – Coconut milk is lactose-free so can be drunk by those who are lactose-intolerant. Go for the 'lighter' lower fat option where you can. Coconut is actually a fruit, not a nut. Nearly all the parts of the fruit can be eaten; the milk, water, flesh, sugar and oil. Even the husks and leaves can be used in furnishings.

MANGO-TASTIC – Mangoes contain a store of phenolic and carotene compounds that seem to offer some protection against some kinds of cancer. Plus, the beta-carotene they contain can boost eye health while vitamin C boosts immunity and the soluble fibre helps to slow down the release of energy from the naturally occurring fruit sugar into the blood.

BLEND **SERVES 1**

¼ medium pineapple, peeled, core left in, cut into chunks

½ small mango, stoned/pitted, peeled, cut into chunks

25g/1oz/1 cup shredded kale

50g/2oz/2 broccoli florets, quartered

1cm/½in piece fresh root ginger, no need to peel, halved

125ml/4fl oz/½ cup canned light coconut milk

175ml/6fl oz/¾ cup water

Energy 177kcal/758kJ; Protein 4.8g; Carbohydrate 38.1g, of which sugars 37.8g; Fat 1.8g, of which saturates 0.5g; Cholesterol 0mg; Calcium 142mg; Fibre 8.6g; Sodium 158mg.

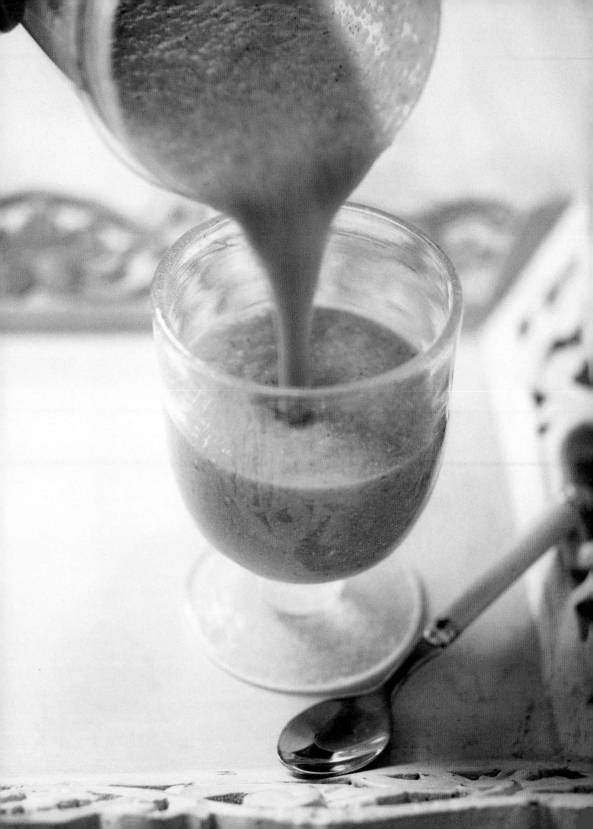

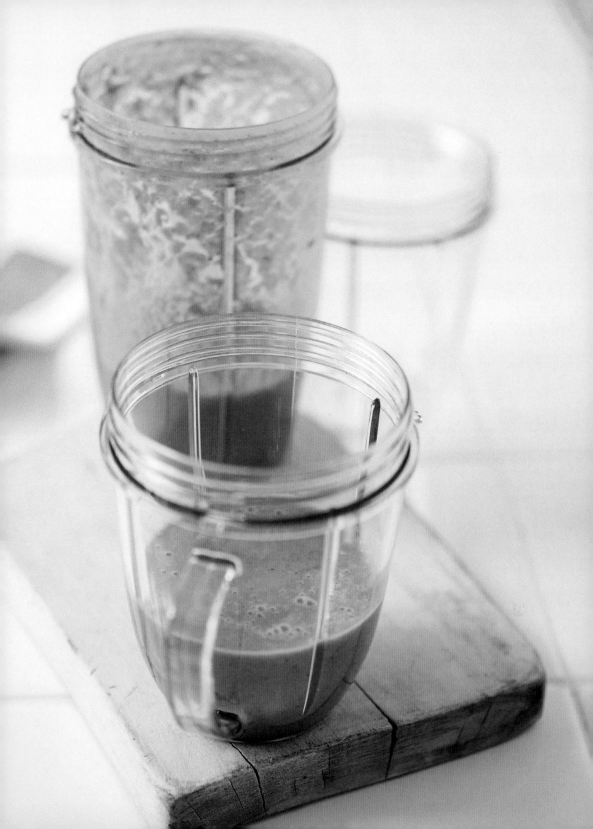

Green giant

This thick, filling and sustaining smoothie really is a meal in a glass and a much healthier option than a caffeine- and calorie-laden cappuccino-style coffee.

1 Add the kiwi fruit, avocado, spinach and kale leaves to a blender goblet. Spoon in the protein powder and camu camu powder. Pour in the coconut water, secure the lid and blitz until smooth.

2 If your blender goblet is small then add just half the coconut water and blitz together until smooth, then add the remaining coconut water and blitz until smooth once more. Pour into a tall glass and serve.

SUPERFOOD NOTE – More than half the calories in an avocado come from the world's healthiest fat – monounsaturated fat, which boosts energy levels and some research suggests may improve your cholesterol profile. Omega 9 fats help reduce skin redness and irritation and the antioxidant carotenoids E and C may also help hold back the signs of skin ageing.

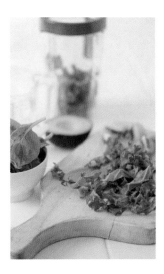

BLEND SERVES 1

1 kiwi fruit, peeled, cut into chunks

½ small avocado, stoned/pitted, flesh scooped from skin

15g/½oz/½ cup baby spinach leaves

15g/½oz/½ cup shredded kale

10ml/2 tsp unflavoured pea protein powder

2.5ml/½ tsp camu camu powder

250ml/8fl oz/1 cup coconut water from a carton, or water

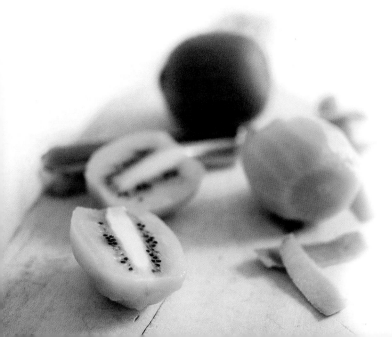

Energy 216kcal/899kJ; Protein 11.2g; Carbohydrate 8.6g, of which sugars 7g; Fat 15.5g, of which saturates 3.1g; Cholesterol 0mg; Calcium 68mg; Fibre 6.3g; Sodium 34mg.

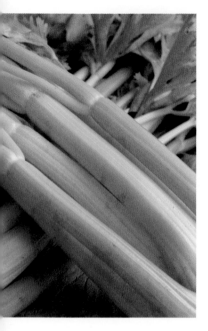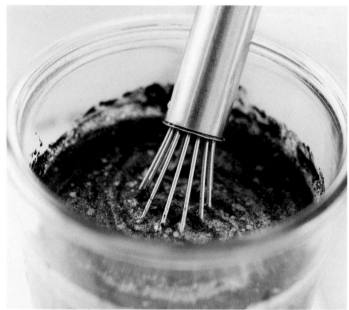

Zingy refresher

JUICE **SERVES 1**

50g/2oz/2 cups/2 handfuls
baby spinach leaves

¼ medium pineapple,
skin cut away, core left in,
halved lengthways

½ cucumber

2 sticks celery

5cm/2in piece broccoli stalk

1.5–2.5ml/¼–½ tsp spirulina
powder

Spirulina transforms this mid-green juice into the most dramatic dark green. Rich in protein and Vitamin B12 – a vitamin that can be difficult to obtain in sufficient amounts on a vegetarian diet – plus calcium and iron, it's the high levels of chlorophyll that makes the colour so intense. Sold in powdered form it makes a handy store-cupboard superfood booster to this refreshing and thirst-quenching breakfast drink.

1 Gradually press all the vegetables and fruit through the juicer. Add the spirulina powder to the juice to taste, and whisk together until smooth.

2 Pour into a glass and serve.

COOK'S TIP – Don't throw broccoli stems away, keep them to add to green juices. They have just as many nutrients as the florets.

Energy 117kcal/496kJ; Protein 4.3g; Carbohydrate 23.5g, of which sugars 23.3g; Fat 1.2g, of which saturates 0.1g; Cholesterol 0mg; Calcium 178mg; Fibre 1.2g; Sodium 115mg.

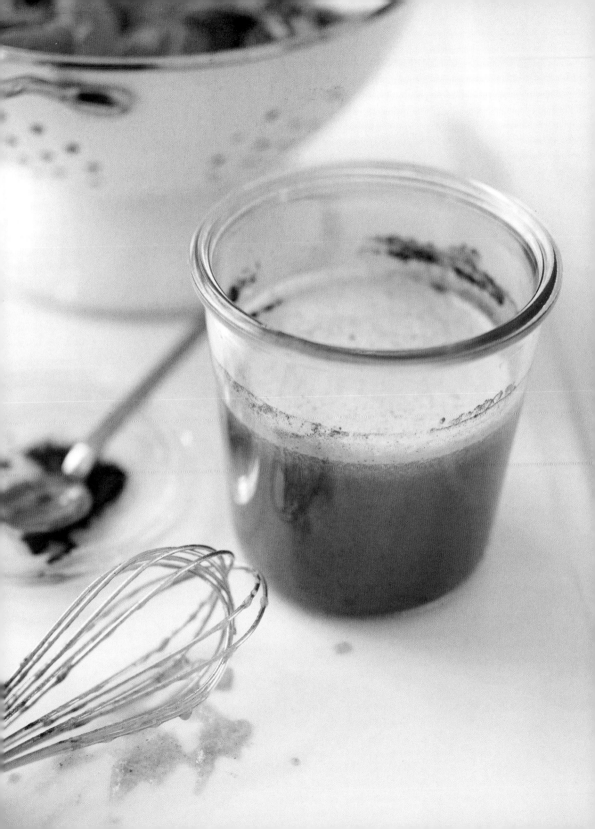

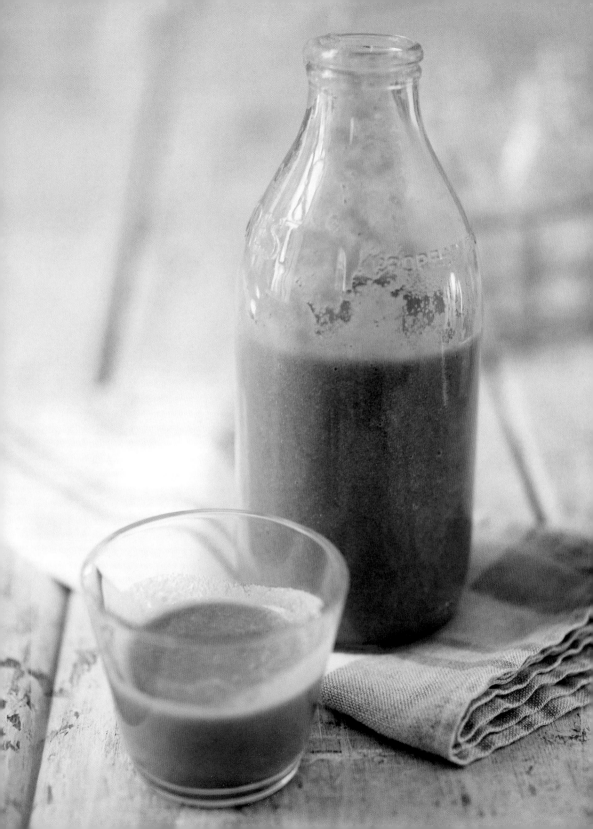

Cauliflower jumpstart

Cauliflowers are back in fashion and now high on the superfood list as they contain vitamins, minerals, antioxidants and phytochemicals. While they may not be the obvious choice for a shake-style drink they add a creamy smoothness that combines with the natural sweetness of the banana and earthy flavour of the mushroom tea, in this energizing breakfast-boosting combo.

1 Add the mushroom tea powder and boiling water to a cup and mix together until all the powder has dissolved. Pour into a blender goblet then add the cauliflower, banana, courgette, spinach and broccoli.

2 Pour in the water, secure the lid and blitz until smooth and frothy. Stir in the maple syrup or sweetener of choice to taste and pour into a glass to serve.

CANCER-FIGHTING – Cauliflower contains sulforaphane, thought by some researchers to help slow the growth of some cancers.

BLEND SERVES 1

1 sachet or 5ml/1 tsp powdered instant chaga mushroom tea

50ml/2fl oz/¼ cup boiling water

¼ small cauliflower with a few tiny attached leaves, cut into chunks

1 small banana, cut into chunks

75g/3oz courgette/zucchini, sliced

25g/1oz/1 cup/1 handful baby spinach leaves

50g/2oz broccoli florets

175ml/6fl oz/½ cup cold water

5ml/1 tsp maple syrup or sweetener of choice

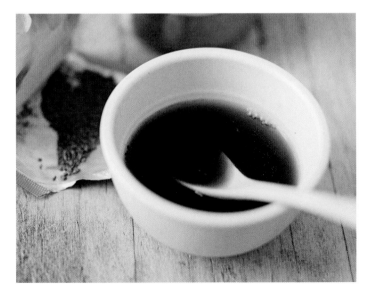

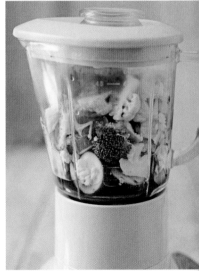

Energy 168kcal/705kJ; Protein 9.7g; Carbohydrate 28.3g, of which sugars 25.3g; Fat 2.3g, of which saturates 0.5g; Cholesterol 0mg; Calcium 124mg; Fibre 7.5g; Sodium 52mg.

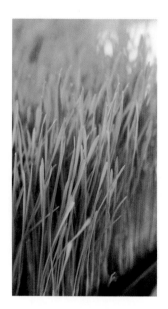

Swiss mix

All the flavours of a classic Bircher muesli mixed with goji berries, wheatgrass and kale for a modern twist on a favourite healthy breakfast.

1 Add all the ingredients to a blender goblet, add the lid and blitz until smooth. Pour into a glass and serve.

GO GOJI GO – These tiny dried red berries are now widely available in supermarkets and health food stores. They are rich in carotenes which help to boost our immune system, and some research suggests that regular consumption may protect against heart disease and cancer.

COOK'S TIP – If you don't have any oat milk then use unsweetened almond or rice milk instead.

BLEND **SERVES 1**

15ml/1 tbsp rolled oats

6 unblanched almonds

15ml/1 tbsp sunflower seeds

15ml/1 tbsp dried
goji berries

5ml/1 tsp wheatgrass powder

1 kiwi fruit, peeled,
cut into chunks

½ pear, no need to peel,
cut into chunks

25g/1oz/1 cup/1 handful
shredded kale

250ml/8fl oz/1 cup
unsweetened oat milk

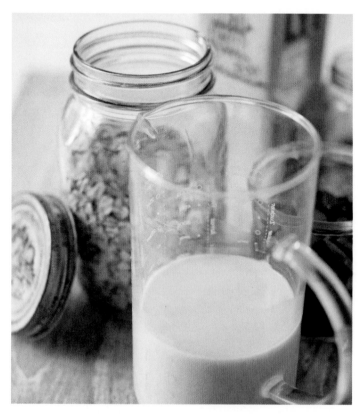

Energy 653kcal/1918kJ; Protein 12.4g; Carbohydrate 42.7g, of which sugars 33.9g; Fat 20.7g, of which saturates 1.7g; Cholesterol 0mg; Calcium 116mg; Fibre 7.7g; Sodium 23mg.

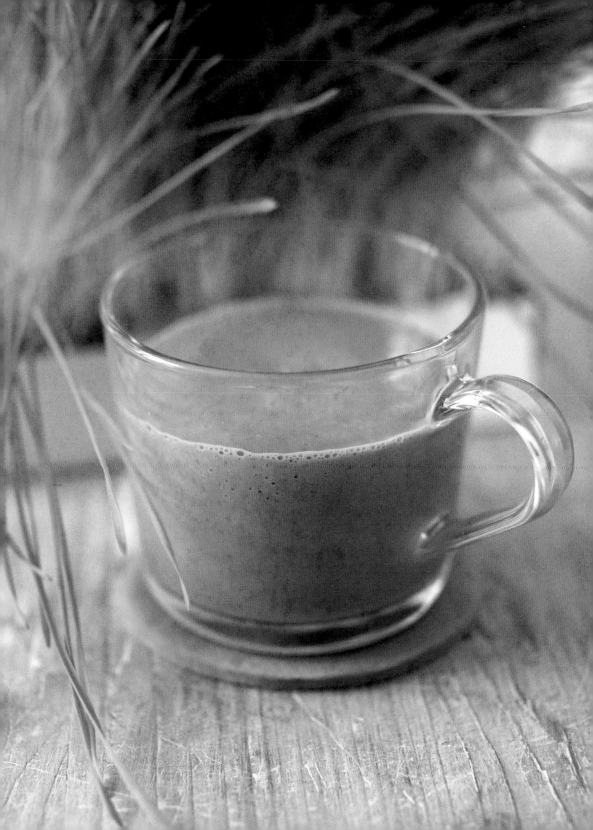

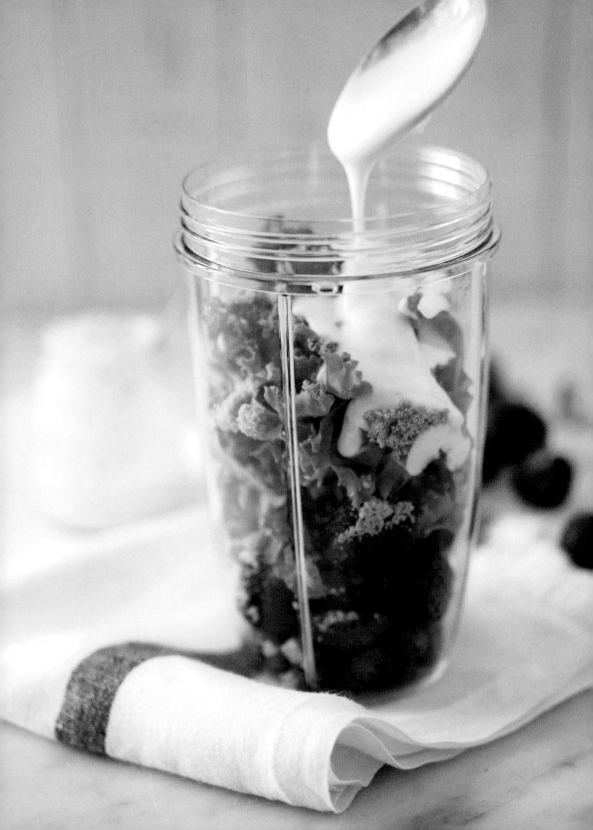

Vitamin C supercharge

Rich in vitamin C, berries and kale help the white blood cells fight infections, so boosting immunity, and if that wasn't enough, they help to keep our skin youthful by producing collagen, a type of protein that maintains the skins elasticity. Who needs expensive face creams!

1 Add all the ingredients to a blender goblet, add the lid and blitz until smooth and frothy. Stir in a little extra water if needed then pour into a tall glass.

SUPERFOOD NOTE – Blueberries make a fantastic fruit choice, naturally sweet but just 57 calories per 100g/4oz. They are packed with nutrients – vitamins C, A and E – which together work as potent antioxidants, plus phenol compounds and fibre for optimum health.
NUTRIENT NOTE –Yogurt contains naturally produced cultures or probiotics, the good bacteria that help maintain a healthy gut and immune system. Its mild creamy soothing taste is also said to help reduce bad breath too.
COOK'S TIP – Choose fresh berries in summer when their flavour is at their best. During the winter months when prices are high, frozen make a great standby; just take out as many as and when you need, and blitz while still frozen.

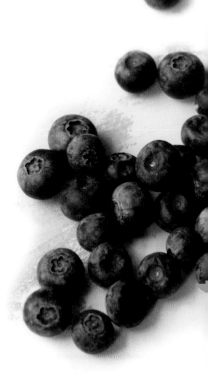

BLEND SERVES 1

25g/1oz/1 cup shredded kale

50g/2oz/½ cup blueberries

75g/3oz or 3 strawberries, hulled, halved or quartered

115g/4oz/½ cup low-fat plain yogurt or non-dairy alternative

15ml/1 tbsp ground seed mix, see left

125ml/4fl oz/½ cup water, or to taste

GROUND SEED MIX
Makes 125g/4¼oz/
generous 1 cup:
Add 45ml/3 tbsp each of sesame, sunflower, pumpkin and golden flaxseeds to a blender goblet or spice mill, and blend until finely ground. Scoop out and store in a sealed plastic container in the refrigerator for up to 2 weeks.

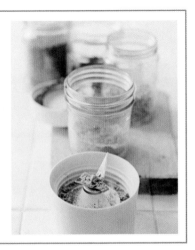

Energy 209kcal/875kJ; Protein 9.9g; Carbohydrate 23.8g, of which sugars 19g; Fat 8.9g, of which saturates 1.8g; Cholesterol 2mg; Calcium 247mg; Fibre 4.9g; Sodium 89mg.

Good morning shake

BLEND SERVES 1

10 unblanched almonds

15ml/1 tbsp pumpkin seeds

15ml/1 tbsp unflavoured pea protein or hemp powder

1 ripe pear, quartered, cored, but not peeled, cut into chunks

100g/3¾oz/½ cup seedless green grapes

25g/1oz/1 cup shredded kale

175ml/6fl oz/¾ cup coconut water from a carton

Boost energy levels with naturally sweet high-fibre fruits rather than processed sugary breakfast cereals. There is strong evidence that the natural pectin (the substance that helps jam to set) found in the soluble fibre of pears and apples can help to lower cholesterol in the blood and to slow down the rate at which glucose is absorbed.

1 Add all the ingredients to a liquidizer goblet, add the lid and blitz until smooth. Pour into a tall glass to serve.

PROTEIN-BOOSTING ALMONDS – Almonds are an easy way to provide protein in a shake and for those on a vegetarian diet are good for boosting those vitamins and minerals usually found in animal sources. The unsaturated fats they contain boost energy.

NUTRIENT NOTE – Coconut water is a naturally clear liquid taken from young green coconuts, it has less calories than coconut milk and more potassium than a sports drink. It is super-hydrating with a slightly nutty taste.

COOK'S TIP – Pea protein powder or hemp powder is a great way for those on a vegan diet to boost protein levels. Buy plain or flavoured from the health food store.

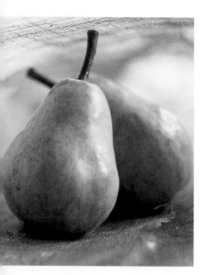

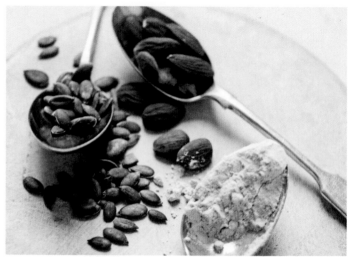

Energy 573kcal/2393kJ; Protein 28.2g; Carbohydrate 37g, of which sugars 33g; Fat 35.6g, of which saturates 3.3g; Cholesterol 0mg; Calcium 188mg; Fibre 7.9g; Sodium 27mg.

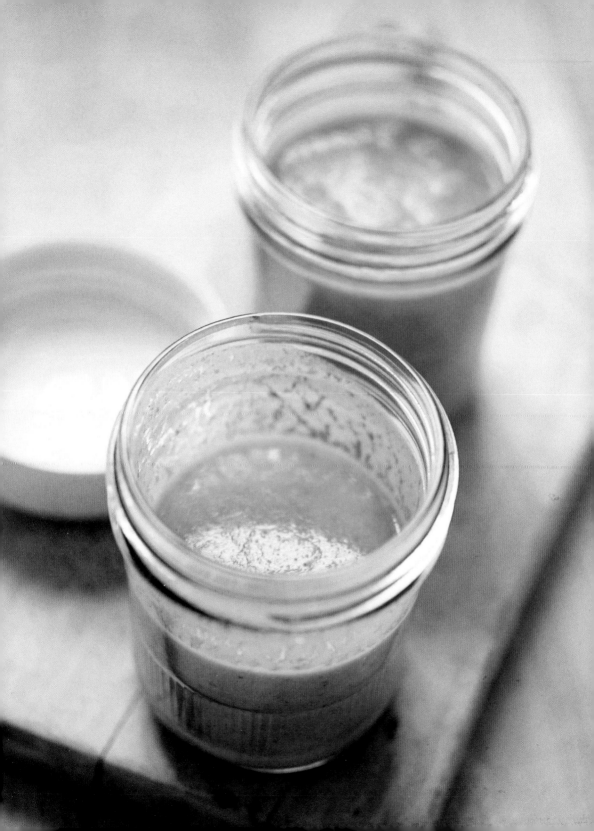

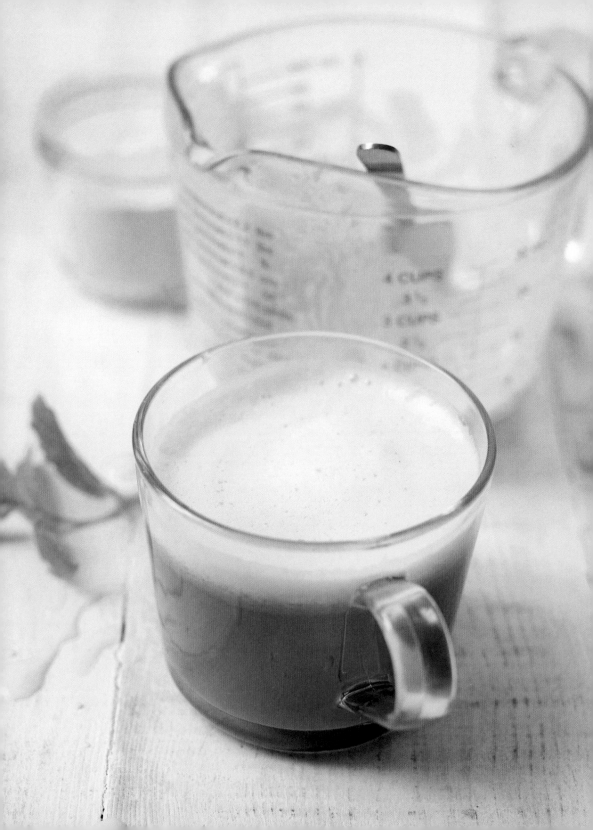

Wake-up call

Awaken those tastebuds with this refreshing, zingy, pretty pale green juice. Cucumber aids hydration, while the green grapes add natural sweetness and mint aids digestion.

1 Add the rocket leaves to the juicer chute then gradually press all the remaining ingredients through the juicer except the baobab powder. Whisk in the baobab powder, if using, and pour into a glass to serve.

GO GREEN – Green apples contain the natural setting agent pectin which helps to remove excess cholesterol from the digestive tract and helps to stimulate the growth of healthy bacteria in the large intestine.

NUTRIENT NOTE – Water is just as important as nutrients in the diet to keep our body hydrated and to help you stay focussed and able to concentrate. We should aim to drink 1.75 litres/3 pints of water a day but this can be a mix of water, freshly made juices, fruit teas, decaffeinated tea and coffee and water.

COOK'S TIP – Baobab powder can be bought from any good health food store. It is rich in probiotics plus potassium, calcium, magnesium and vitamin C.

JUICE **SERVES 1**

25g/1oz/1 cup rocket/ arugula leaves

25g/1oz/1 cup baby spinach leaves

3 stems fresh mint

1 green apple

½ cucumber

75g/3oz/½ cup seedless green grapes

5ml/1 tsp baobab powder, optional

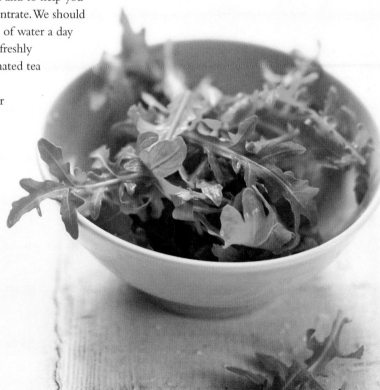

Energy 140kcal/588kJ; Protein 3.6g; Carbohydrate 31g, of which sugars 30.8g; Fat 0.8g, of which saturates 0.1g; Cholesterol 0mg; Calcium 138mg; Fibre 1.1g; Sodium 81mg.

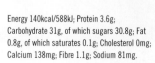

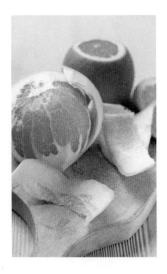

Citrus burst

Light and super-refreshing, this is tea but not as you know it. Grapefruit adds a slight sharpness that wakes you up in a far healthier way than a strong cup of tea or caffeine-loaded black coffee.

1 Press the grapefruit, orange and apple through the juicer then process the lettuce.

2 Pour the juice into a glass, add the tea powder and fork together.

SUPERFOOD NOTE – Matcha green tea is a powdered and concentrated form of green tea leaves and contains 137 times the antioxidants of regular green tea.

JUICE **SERVES 1**

1 white-fleshed grapefruit, peel and pith cut away

1 orange, peel and pith cut away

1 green apple

½ romaine lettuce

2.5ml/½ tsp Matcha green tea powder

Energy 94kcal/398kJ; Protein 2.7g; Carbohydrate 21.2g, of which sugars 21.2g; Fat 0.3g, of which saturates 0g; Cholesterol 0mg; Calcium 95mg; Fibre 1.0g; Sodium 11mg.

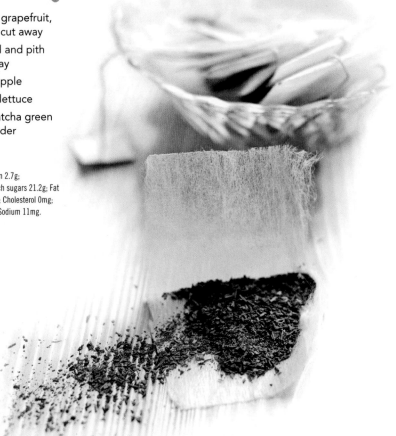

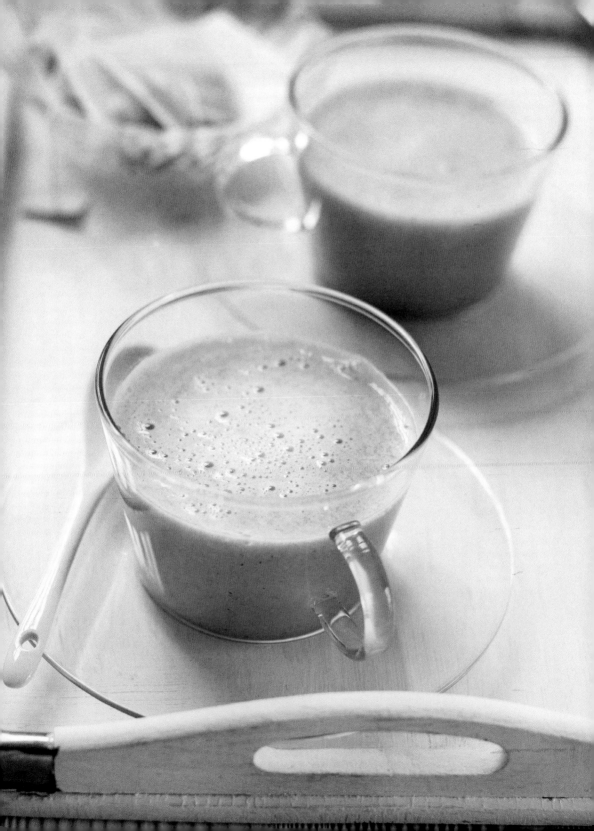

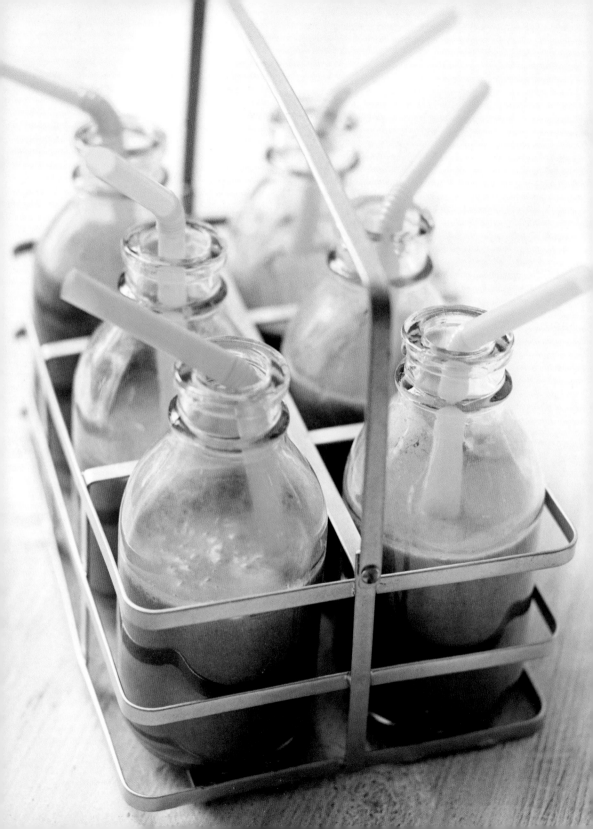

Cacao comforter

You don't need to miss out on a chocolate fix when trying to eat in a healthier way. This super-filling, energy-boosting meal in a glass will sustain you until lunchtime. Mixing raw cacao powder with kale is a good way to tempt those sceptics who say kale isn't for them.

1 Add all the ingredients to a blender goblet, add the lid and blitz until smooth and frothy. Adjust the consistency with a little water or extra almond milk if needed then pour into a tall glass to serve.

SUPERFOOD NOTE – Bananas are the most popular fruit in the world and grown in more than 150 countries. A medium-sized banana contains just 95 calories for a quick but sustained energy boost in a natural, nutritious and easily digestible form.

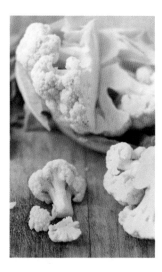

BLEND SERVES 1

10ml/2 tsp raw cacao powder

pinch ground cinnamon

250ml/8fl oz/1 cup
unsweetened almond milk

50g/2oz or 3 cauliflower
florets

25g/1oz/1 cup/1 handful
shredded kale

25g/1oz or 1 large date,
stoned/pitted

½ banana

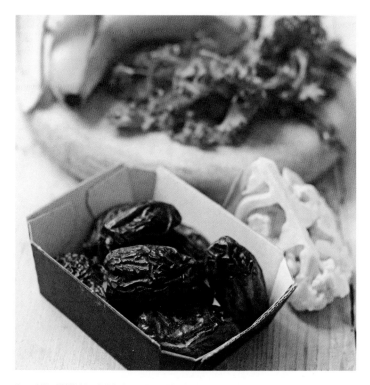

Energy 242kcal/1023kJ; Protein 6.5g; Carbohydrate 47.7g, of which sugars 44.7g; Fat 4.2g, of which saturates 0.8g; Cholesterol 0mg; Calcium 65mg; Fibre 5.7g; Sodium 223mg.

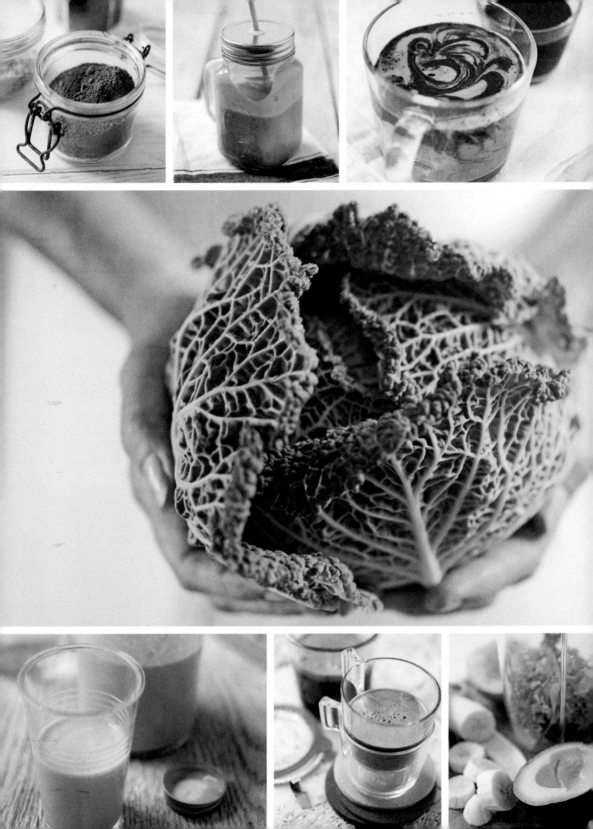

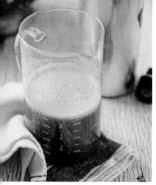

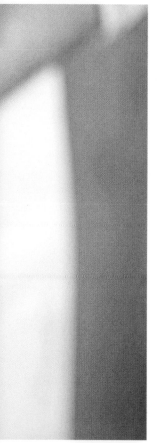

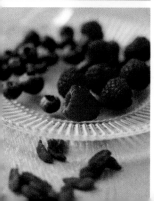

ENERGY-BOOSTERS

We all need an energy boost at some point during the day, perhaps before or after an exercise class or run, to keep you on top form in a pressurized job, or to cope with the stresses and strains of being a busy parent with a demanding family. Made with avocados, bananas, papaya and beetroot these drinks are higher in energy-boosting carbs and calories but also provide all-important slow-release energy to fight fatigue and maintain concentration levels.

Super-powered berry bonanza

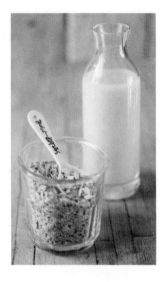

Don't reach for the quick sugary, energy-boosting biscuits or cake. Slow-release carbs in the form of oats, berries, kale and banana make for a much healthier option as they help to stabilize blood sugar levels but also contain vital vitamins and minerals to keep us in top shape.

1 Add the berries to a blender goblet, or if you have a smaller second blender goblet, use this. Add the lid and blitz until smooth. Decant the berry purée into a small bowl – if you only have one blender goblet then rinse out.

2 Blend all the remaining ingredients together until smooth then pour into a tall glass. Spoon the berry purée over the top and swirl together with a teaspoon or leave as an attractive layer as shown.

BLEND **SERVES 1**

75g/3oz/½ cup raspberries

75g/3oz/½ cup blueberries or blackberries

30ml/2 tbsp rolled oats

50g/2oz or 3 romaine lettuce leaves, torn into pieces

25g/1oz/1 cup shredded kale

½ banana, sliced

10ml/2 tsp dried goji berries

250ml/8fl oz/1 cup oat milk

CALMING BLUEBERRIES – Rich in antioxidants, blueberries may help to stabilize brain function and protect neural tissue from oxidative stress. This may improve memory and learning, and even reduce the symptoms of depression.

NUTRIENT NOTE – Oats are not only rich in slow-release energy but the soluble fibre they contain also helps lower blood cholesterol. Low in fat, they also contain the protein avenin, which is similar to gluten but can be tolerated by some people sensitive to gluten. (Check with your medical practitioner before introducing into your diet if you are a coeliac, and always check the pack details to check they are gluten-free. Oats can become contaminated with gluten during harvesting, milling or transportation.)

COOK'S TIP – Frozen berries make a handy standby; simply take out a handful as and when you need them. Add them straight from the freezer as a fruity ice cube alternative.

Energy 494kcal/1539kJ; Protein 9.1g; Carbohydrate 51.6g, of which sugars 35.3g; Fat 6.8g, of which saturates 0.3g; Cholesterol 0mg; Calcium 73mg; Fibre 9.9g; Sodium 16mg.

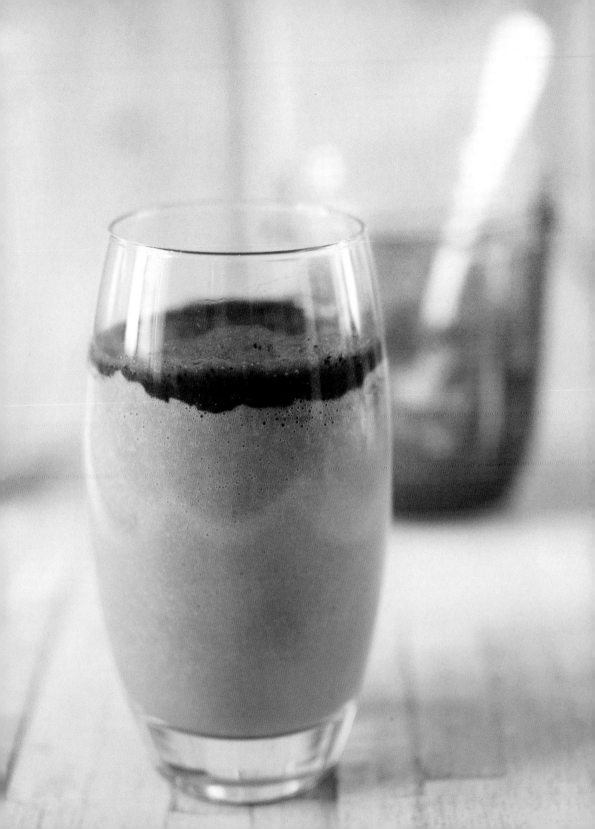

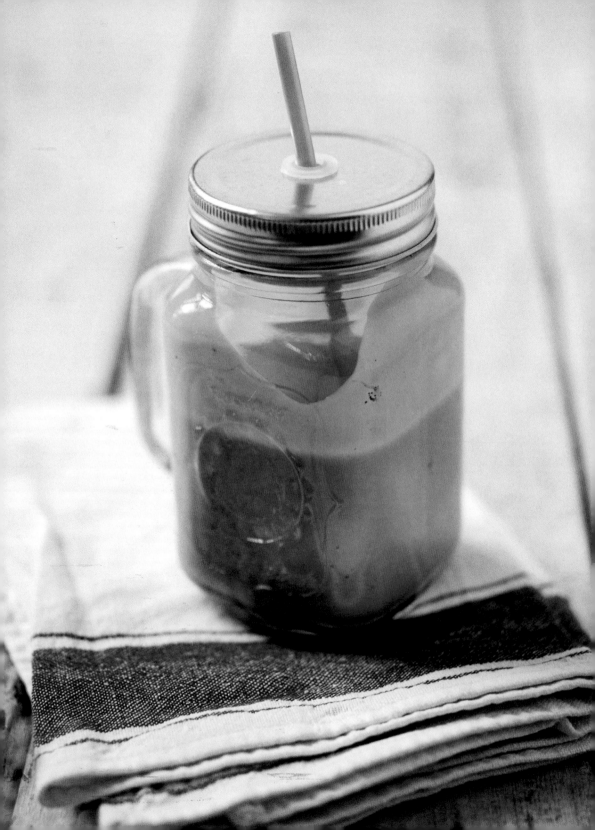

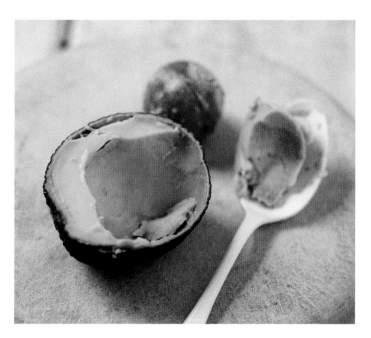

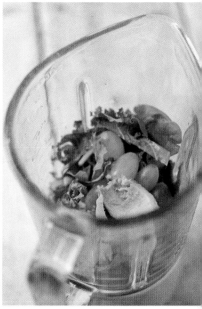

Green tornado

Bursting with complex carbs and natural fruit sugars, this velvety smooth nutrient-bursting tornado of a smoothie will superpower you through any sporting activity or boost energy levels post exercise.

1 Add the kale, spinach, grapes and avocado to the blender goblet then pour in the coconut water, add the lid and blitz until smooth. Add the ice cubes and blitz again until crushed.

2 Pour into a tall glass and stir in lime juice to taste.

FIGHT FATIGUE – Dark green kale and spinach are rich in chlorophyll which helps the blood with oxygenation, health and replenishment of red blood cells, so boosting energy levels and combatting tiredness.

COOK'S TIP – Having a ripe avocado is essential for this smoothie. If it is under-ripe you won't be able to get a really smooth texture.

BLEND SERVES 1

15g/½oz/½ cup shredded kale

25g/1oz baby spinach leaves

100g/4oz/1 cup green seedless grapes

½ ripe avocado, stoned/pitted, flesh scooped from shell

250ml/8fl oz/1 cup coconut water from a carton

few ice cubes

juice of ½ lime

Energy 261kcal/1088kJ; Protein 3.5g; Carbohydrate 17.9g, of which sugars 16.5g; Fat 20g, of which saturates 4.2g; Cholesterol 0mg; Calcium 86mg; Fibre 6.8g; Sodium 49mg.

Cacao and avocado smoothie

BLEND **SERVES 1**

10ml/2 tsp raw cacao powder

10ml/2 tsp dried goji berries

15ml/1 tbsp ground seed mix, see p47

½ ripe avocado, stoned/ pitted, flesh scooped from skin

½ small banana, sliced

½ orange, freshly squeezed juice and flesh scraped from shell

25g/1oz/1 cup shredded kale

125ml/4fl oz/½ cup canned light coconut milk

125ml/4fl oz/½ cup water

A rich chocolatey hit with a smooth velvety texture that will leave you feeling re-energized and raring to go.

1 Add all the ingredients to the blender goblet, secure the lid and blitz until smooth. Pour into a tall glass and serve.

GOOD FATS – Avocados and coconut milk contain fat but they are good fats. While we should watch the kinds of fat that we eat and avoid deep fried foods or saturated fats, we still need fat for every cell in our body; it insulates us from heat loss, cushions vital organs and provides essential fatty acids as well as aiding the absorption of essential fat-soluble vitamins. Weight-for-weight fat provides three times as much energy as carbohydrates.

NUTRIENT TIP – Mixed seeds are a great way to boost protein, vitamin and mineral levels. So that the body can absorb as much of their nutritional value as possible, grind them before eating.

COOK'S TIP – Oranges kept at room temperature are not only easier to squeeze but you will get more juice out of them.

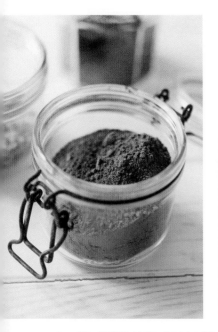
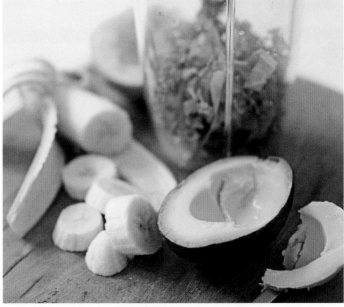

Energy 556kcal/1778kJ; Protein 10.1g; Carbohydrate 33.9g, of which sugars 27.2g; Fat 31.7g, of which saturates 7.9g; Cholesterol 0mg; Calcium 224mg; Fibre 11.1g; Sodium 253mg.

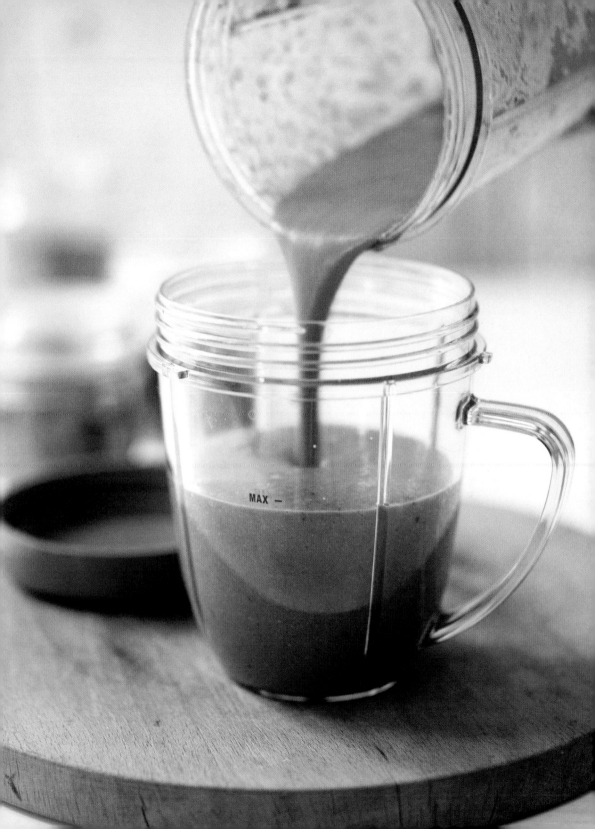

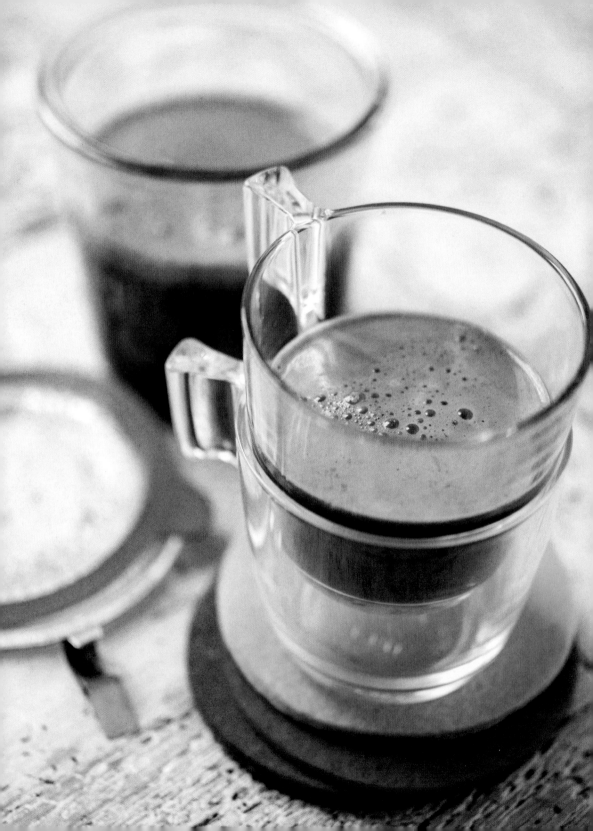

Citrus beet blast

After exercise you not only lose water but minerals through sweat. Rehydration is key but it is also important to boost mineral and energy levels too, to aid recovery time. Packed with concentrated goodness, this is one super-charged juice.

1 Pack the spinach into the feeder chute of the juicer then gradually press all the remaining fruit and vegetables through. Stir the water into the juice, pour into a glass and sweeten to taste.

BEETROOT, THE ATHLETE'S CHOICE – Naturally sweet beetroot contains the equivalent of 5ml/1 tsp of sugar per 100g/4oz, so this juice is a great way to boost energy levels, plus it contains folates, vitamin C, iron and potassium which helps to regulate blood pressure and nerve function. The high levels of nitrates have been shown to benefit cyclists and marathon runners before a race, to sustain them and keep them energized over long distances. Just make sure to take it to events in a well-sealed container!

NUTRIENT NOTE – The brighter or stronger the coloured fruit and vegetables, the more antioxidant vitamins and minerals they contain. Antioxidants are believed to help prevent free-radical damage in the body, which can lead to cancer.

COOK'S TIP – A small handful of shredded green kale can be used in place of the cavolo nero if preferred.

JUICE **SERVES 1**

25g/1oz/1 cup baby spinach

3 cavolo nero or black kale leaves

1 green apple

1 carrot

1 small beetroot/beet, trimmed

½ large orange, peel and pith cut away

175ml/6fl oz/¾ cup water

5ml/1 tsp honey, maple syrup or sweetener of choice

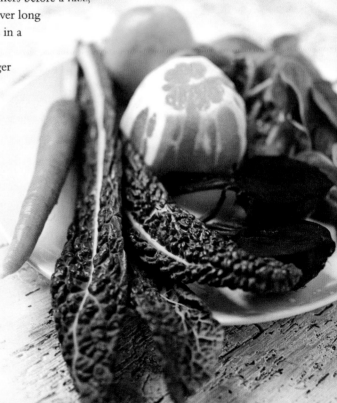

Energy 112kcal/474kJ; Protein 4.7g; Carbohydrate 21.9g, of which sugars 21.8g; Fat 1.2g, of which saturates 0.1g; Cholesterol 0mg; Calcium 259mg; Fibre 0.9g; Sodium 230mg.

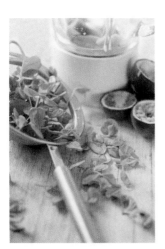

Papaya passion

Just half a papaya provides an adult's daily allowance of vitamin C, not only needed to boost immunity but to produce collagen vital for muscle strength, healthy skin and bones and to stimulate production of white blood cells to help fight infection. Its creamy delicate-tasting flesh adds a wonderful velvety smoothness to this shake.

1 Add all the ingredients to a blender goblet, secure the lid and blitz until smooth. Pour into a tall glass to serve.

ADD A LITTLE PASSION TO YOUR LIFE — Passion fruit pulp is a powerhouse of minerals, including potassium to help regulate the heart rate and blood pressure. It also contains iron, copper, magnesium and phosphorus, not to mention large amounts of vitamins C and A, and lots of soluble fibre to help lower cholesterol and maintain a healthy digestive tract.

BLEND **SERVES 1**

½ papaya, seeds discarded, peeled, flesh cut into chunks

2 passion fruits, halved, pulp and seeds scooped out, shell discarded

15g/½oz/¾ cup pea shoots

30ml/2 tbsp desiccated/ dry unsweetened shredded coconut

125ml/4fl oz/½ cup plain low-fat or non-dairy yogurt

125ml/4fl oz/½ cup coconut water from a carton

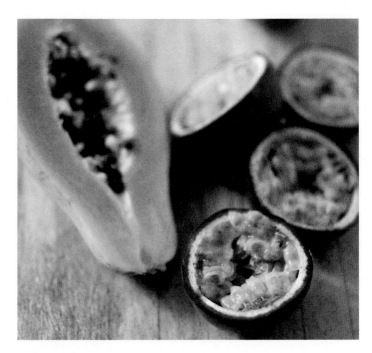

Energy 414kcal/1738kJ; Protein 10.7g; Carbohydrate 49.9g, of which sugars 49.8g; Fat 20.5g, of which saturates 16.9g; Cholesterol 2mg; Calcium 327mg; Fibre 19.5g; Sodium 132mg.

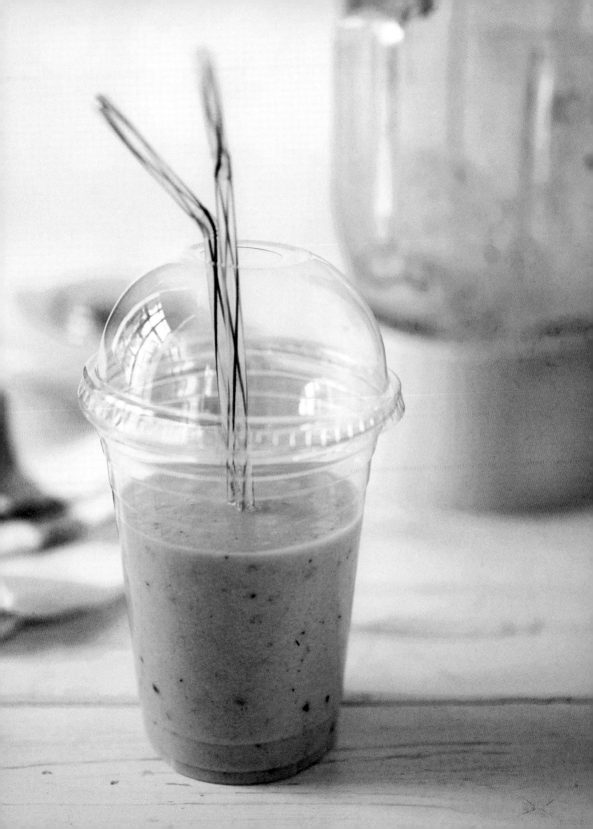

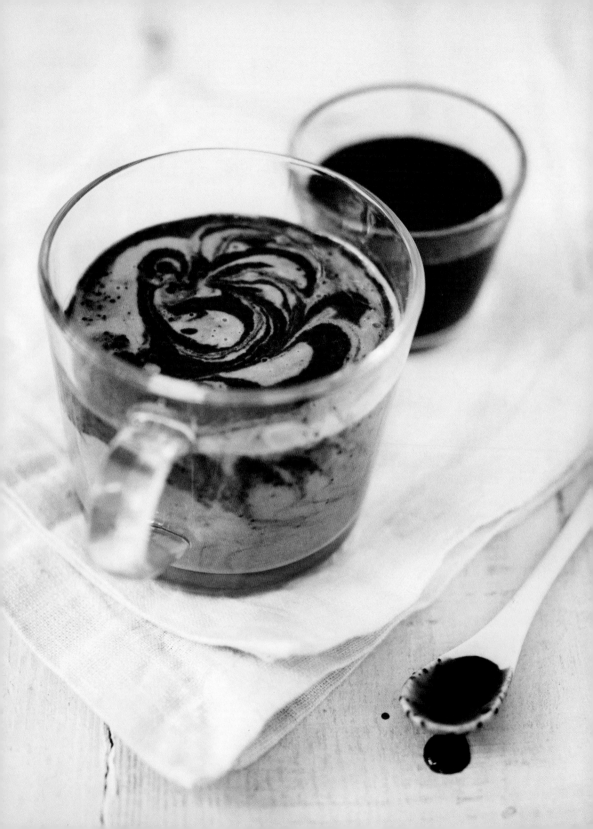

High performance blueberry and kale

Mild, smooth and super-filling. While this may not be the greenest-coloured shake in the book it is full of energy-boosting carbs and healthy fibre, antioxidants, vitamins and minerals for slow sustained release to keep you motivated and on target.

1 Add the blueberries, blackberries and yogurt to a small liquidizer goblet if you have one and blitz until smooth. If you only have one goblet with your machine, decant the purée into a bowl and rinse out.

2 Blend all the remaining ingredients except the sweetener until smooth. Pour into a tall glass, sweeten to taste and adjust the consistency with a little extra water if needed. Pour into a glass and drizzle the berry purée over the top.

NUTRIENT NOTE – When you first start juicing and smoothie-making you will want to add a little honey or sweetener of your choice to this shake, but as you make more and more you will find that your yearning for sweet things will begin to diminish and you will get to the stage when the natural fruit sugars are more than enough. COOK'S TIP – Blueberries last well in the refrigerator but blackberries tend to go soft very quickly. Keep a handy supply of blackberries in the freezer, then just take out a small handful when you need them, and add while still frozen for an instant way to chill your shake.

BLEND SERVES 1

75g/3oz/½ cup blueberries

40g/1½oz/¼ cup fresh or frozen blackberries

45ml/4 tbsp plain low-fat or non-dairy yogurt

15g/½oz/½ cup shredded kale

½ avocado, stoned, flesh scooped from the shell

75g/3oz/¾ cup seedless green grapes

5ml/1 tsp hemp powder

10ml/2 tsp sunflower seeds

250ml/8fl oz/1 cup water

5ml/1 tsp honey or sweetener of choice

Energy 281kcal/1175kJ; Protein 6.3g; Carbohydrate 31.3g, of which sugars 25.5g; Fat 15.6g, of which saturates 3g; Cholesterol 1mg; Calcium 135mg; Fibre 8.4g; Sodium 41mg.

Stamina maximizer

BLEND SERVES 1

½ avocado, stoned/pitted, flesh scooped from shell with a spoon

½ small papaya, seeds discarded, peeled, cut into chunks

25g/1oz/1 cup baby spinach leaves

10 unblanched almonds

10ml/2 tsp ground seed mix, see p47, or ground flaxseeds

250ml/8fl oz/1 cup unsweetened almond milk

125ml/4fl oz/½ cup water

juice of ½ lime

5ml/1 tsp honey (optional)

Thick, creamy and super-satisfying, this pale green avocado and papaya shake will provide slowly released energy to power you through any sporting activity or help boost concentration levels and keep you on target if stuck at your desk.

1 Add the avocado and papaya to the blender goblet then add the spinach, nuts and seeds. Pour in the almond milk, secure the lid and blitz until smooth.

2 Adjust the consistency to taste with water then stir in lime juice and honey to taste, if using. Pour into a tall glass to serve.

ENERGY EFFICIENCY – Even at rest, our brain uses 50% of the energy that is derived from the food that we consume, and considerably more when we engage our brain when working or sitting an exam or doing a sporting activity. During periods of stress we use up even more energy. We get energy from carbohydrates, protein and fat, all of which can be found in this smooth blend.

COOK'S TIP – Unsweetened almond milk has been used here but you can substitute rice milk or oat milk or simply add water if preferred.

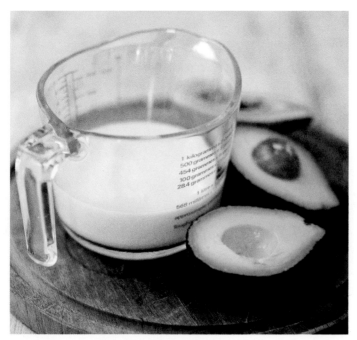

Energy 457kcal/1904kJ; Protein 13.1g; Carbohydrate 32.3g, of which sugars 31g; Fat 31.6g, of which saturates 3g; Cholesterol 0mg; Calcium 252mg; Fibre 7.8g; Sodium 220mg.

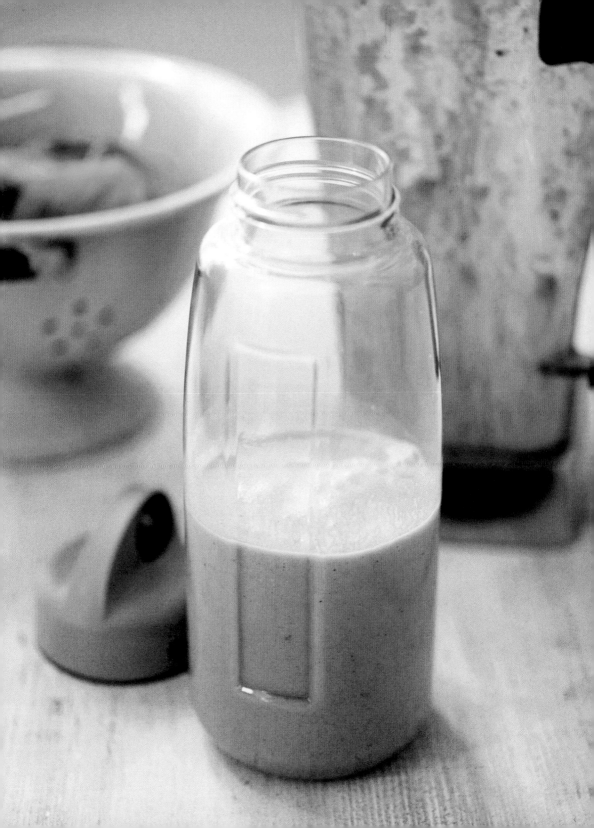

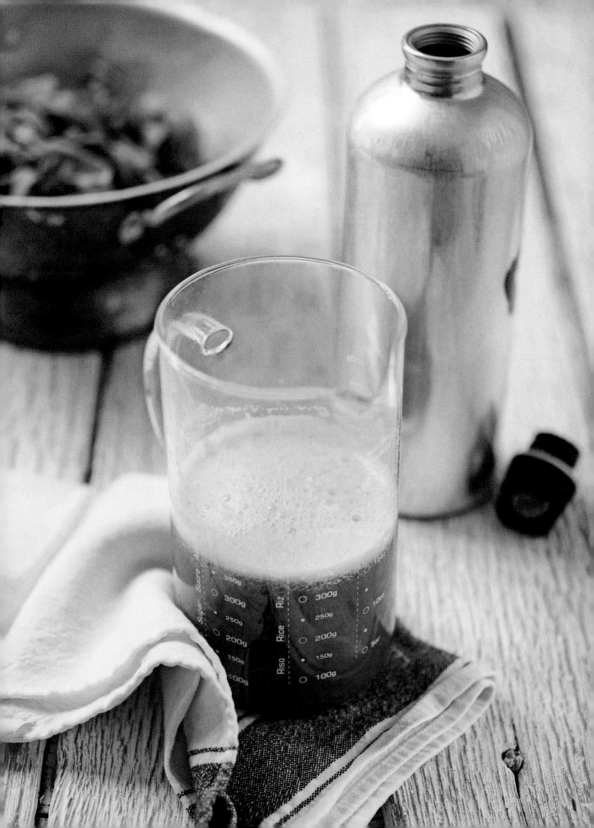

Spinach rejuvenator

Naturally sweet and energizing pear blends well with the vitamin- and mineral-packed spinach and mild-tasting courgette. This is a refreshing, revitalizing and rehydrating mid-morning or mid-afternoon pick-me-up to aid concentration and boost good health.

1 Gradually feed the spinach, courgette and pear through the juicer. Pour into a tall glass and stir in the hemp oil.

SUPER SPINACH – Rich in antioxidants to help reduce the risk of heart disease and cancer, spinach also contains lutein, a carotenoid antioxidant that helps protect against cataracts and macular degeneration.

NUTRIENT NOTE – The pectin in pears helps to lower cholesterol too.

COOK'S TIP – Buy hemp oil in the supermarket (found alongside the olive oil) to boost omega 3 fatty acids in the diet.

JUICE SERVES 1

50g/2oz/2 cups baby spinach leaves

175g/6oz or 1 small courgette/zucchini

1 ripe pear, no need to peel or core

5ml/1 tsp hemp oil

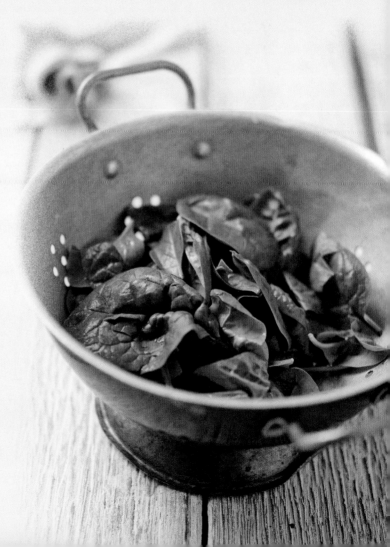

Energy 131kcal/545kJ; Protein 5g; Carbohydrate 18.9g, of which sugars 18.7g; Fat 4.2g, of which saturates 0.7g; Cholesterol 0mg; Calcium 146mg; Fibre 0.7g; Sodium 76mg.

Triple nut combo

BLEND **SERVES 1**

250ml/8fl oz/1 cup unsweetened almond milk

25g/1oz/¼ cup Brazil nuts

25g/1oz/¼ cup hazelnuts

25g/1oz/1 cup baby spinach leaves

1 small banana

few drops vanilla extract

little water or ice, to taste

All the taste and creamy smoothness of a dairy shake, yet this is made with nuts and nut milk for a high-energy, protein and vitamin E-packed drink. The spinach has such a delicate flavour that if it wasn't for the colour you would have no idea that a green vegetable had been added.

1 Add all the ingredients to the blender goblet with the exception of the water. Blitz until really smooth.

2 Add a little water or handful of ice cubes and blitz again until the desired thickness, then pour into a tall glass to serve.

GO BANANAS – Full of complex carbs, bananas boost energy, provide potassium to help regulate blood pressure, and tryptophan and vitamin B6 to increase serotonin, the natural good mood chemical. Plus, they add a creamy smoothness to any shake.

NUTRIENT NOTE – Nuts are packed with protein, an essential part of every cell in our body and needed for growth and repair of everything from muscles and bones to hair and fingernails. Protein also aids digestion, produces antibodies that fight off infection and boosts hormones so that our body works efficiently. Nuts do contain fat but it is the healthy unsaturated fatty acids rather than the saturated fat found in red meat.

COOK'S TIP – If using fresh cut spinach from the garden or farm store make sure to rinse off all traces of soil before use.

Energy 448kcal/1857kJ; Protein 9.7g; Carbohydrate 24.1g, of which sugars 21.8g; Fat 35.4g, of which saturates 5.6g; Cholesterol 0mg; Calcium 124mg; Fibre 5.3g; Sodium 205mg.

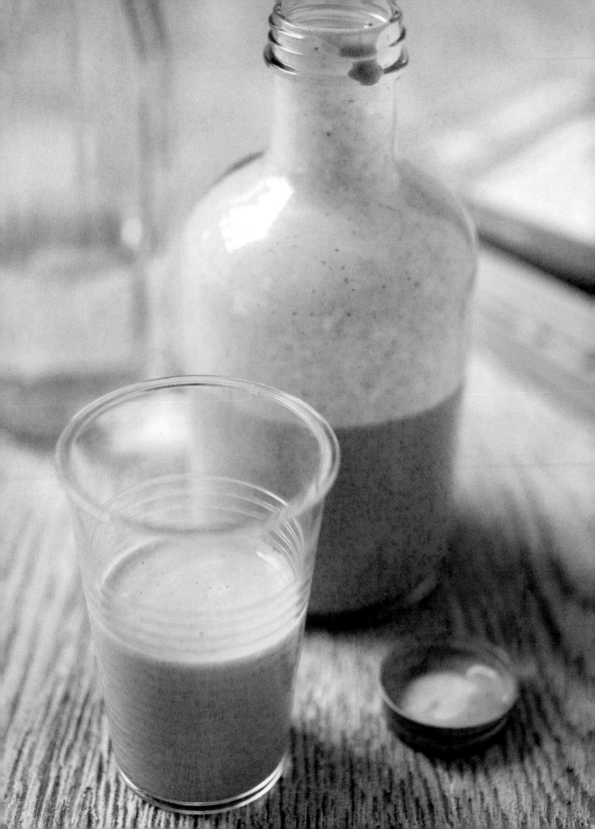

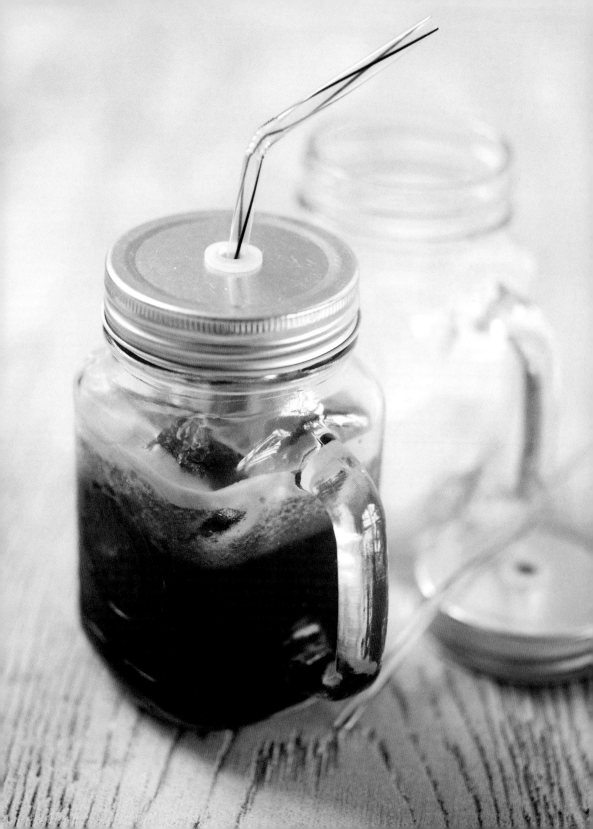

Turbo-charged beet

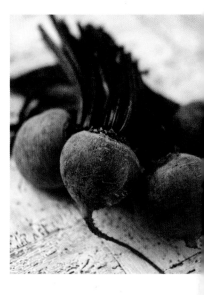

Refuel your body with this tangy, refreshing, homemade isotonic sports drink. Betacyanin is the pigment that gives beetroot its intense colour; if consumed regularly it is thought it may help reduce the oxidation of LDL cholesterol and so help protect artery walls and reduce the risk of heart disease and stroke. It doesn't matter how little beetroot you add to a juice, the finished drink will always be red!

1 Gradually press all the vegetables then fruit through the juicer. Stir in the coconut water then pour into a tall glass half filled with ice cubes, and serve.

WHAT IS AN ISOTONIC DRINK? — These sports drinks replace fluids and electrolytes lost during exercise and are generally made up of glucose, water, vitamins and salts in a similar concentration to your body's own fluids.

JUICE **SERVES 1**

25g/1oz or ½ small trimmed beetroot/beet

50g/2oz/2 cups shredded kale

¼ medium pineapple, peeled, but core left in or 200g/7oz/1 cup prepared pineapple, cut into chunks

1 green apple

125ml/4fl oz/½ cup coconut water from a carton

ice cubes, to serve

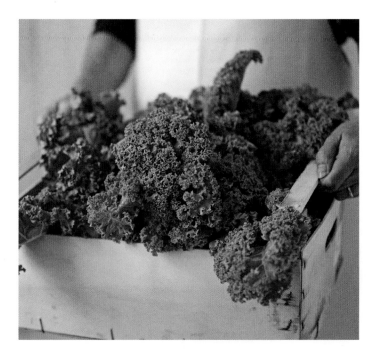

Energy 118kcal/506kJ; Protein 3g; Carbohydrate 25.7g, of which sugars 25.5g; Fat 1.2g, of which saturates 0.1g; Cholesterol 0mg; Calcium 100mg; Fibre 1.3g; Sodium 43mg.

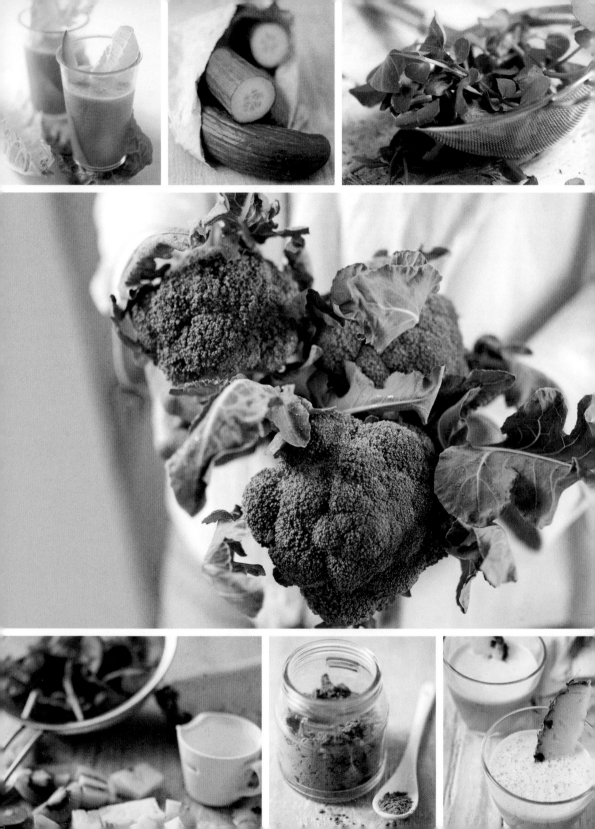

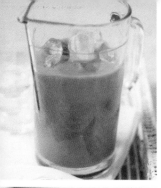

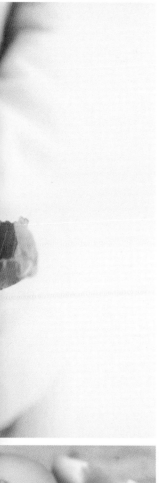

LOW-CALORIE SUPER-JUICES

These reduced-calorie drinks are packed with healthy vegetables and fruit for maximum vitamins and minerals to keep you super-powered, refreshed and alert. Although fruits do contain sugar which will nudge the calorie count up a little, they come mixed with complex carbs and fibre which take the body longer to digest and so help to avoid mood swings.

Super-green vitality

JUICE **SERVES 1**

50g/2oz/2 cups shredded or whole kale leaves

½ cucumber

2 celery sticks

1 ripe pear, no need to peel or core

5ml/1 tsp lacuma powder

5ml/1 tsp hemp powder

A thirst-quenching veggilicious juice rich in cancer-fighting antioxidants, vitamins and minerals but low in calories. The pear adds just a hint of natural sweetness to neutralize and balance the strong taste of kale.

1 Press the kale into the feeder chute of the juicer, then gradually press the cucumber, celery and pear through the juicer.

2 Add the lacuma and hemp powder and fork or whisk together until smooth. Pour into a tall glass and serve.

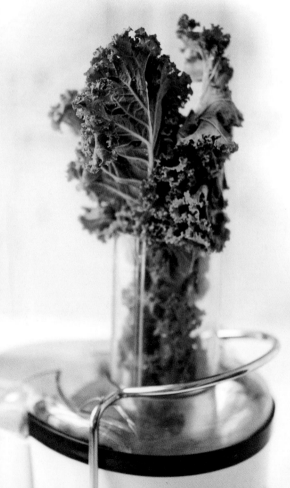

SUPER-HERO KALE – Grown since Roman times, kale is part of the super-healthy cabbage family. Lutein and zeaxanthin give kale its rich, dark colour and may help to slow down macular degeneration and cataracts. It is also rich in the vitamins A, C and K plus a whole range of minerals.

NUTRIENT NOTE – Hemp powder is a high-quality protein that contains all essential amino acids in an easily digested form, making it a great addition to any vegetarian diet. Protein is needed for muscle growth and repair and body maintenance of all cells, tissues and organs. It is also added to non-dairy sports and body-building protein formulas.

COOK'S TIP – Buy pears when a little hard and leave to ripen in a fruit bowl in the kitchen so that the starch they contain turns to sugar, adding flavour. They contain about 70 calories depending on size.

Energy 96kcal/402kJ; Protein 3.5g; Carbohydrate 18.5g, of which sugars 18.3g; Fat 1.2g, of which saturates 0.1g; Cholesterol 0mg; Calcium 133mg; Fibre 0.5g; Sodium 66mg.

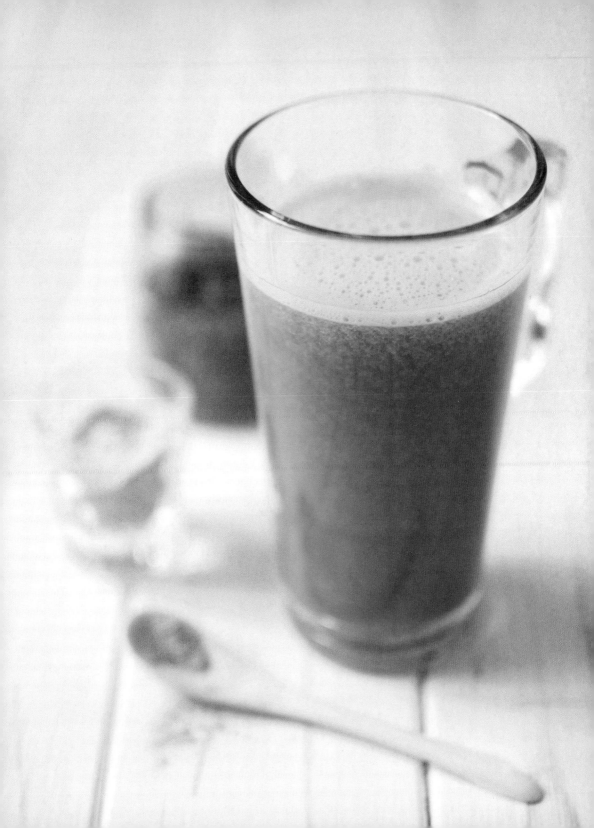

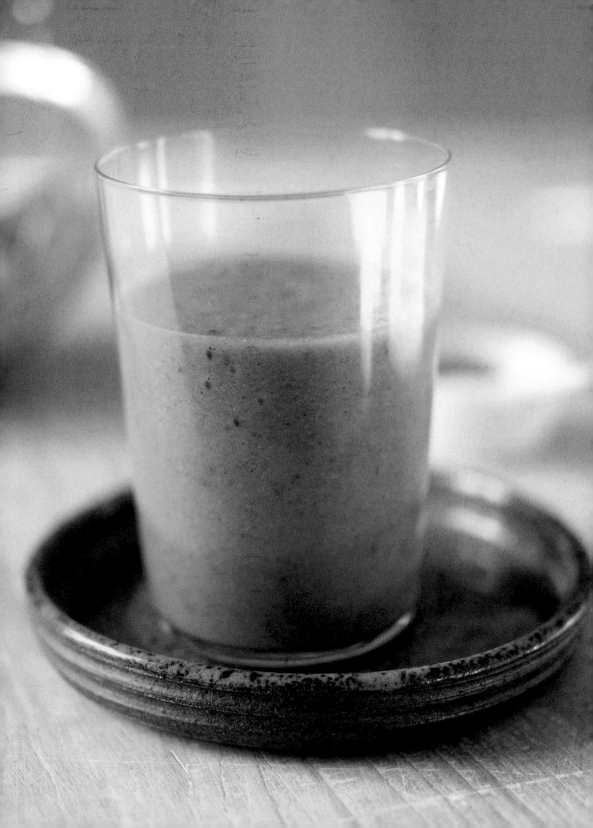

Kiwi reviver

This eye-catching bright green tangy smoothie is speckled with tiny black chia seeds, which are a powerhouse of nutrition – rich in soluble fibre, minerals and omega 3 fatty acids, and beneficial for brain function, lowering inflammation and for cardiovascular health.

1 Add all the ingredients except the chia seeds to a blender goblet, secure the lid and blitz until smooth.

2 Stir in the chia seeds and a little extra water, if needed. Pour into a tall tumbler to serve.

SUPERFOOD NOTE – Kiwi fruit is loaded with nutrition. An excellent source of cancer-fighting antioxidants, large amounts of vitamin C to boost the immune system and fight the effects of stress and aging, plus potassium and fibre.
COOK'S TIP – Chia seeds swell when they come into contact with liquid so drink this as soon as you have made it or you may find you will need a spoon! Once drunk the gelling action in your stomach will give the sensation of feeling fuller for longer, a great aid if you are trying to lose weight.

BLEND SERVES 1

1 kiwi fruit, peeled, roughly chopped

¼ medium pineapple, peeled, core left in, roughly chopped

25g/1oz/1 handful baby spinach leaves

5cm/2in piece cucumber, diced

125ml/4fl oz/½ cup water

5ml/1 tsp chia seeds

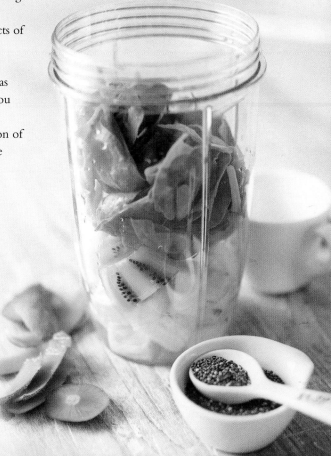

Energy 120kcal/510kJ; Protein 2.3g;
Carbohydrate 27.3g, of which sugars 27g; Fat
0.9g, of which saturates 0g; Cholesterol 0mg;
Calcium 97mg; Fibre 5.6g; Sodium 42mg.

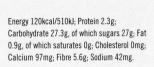

1 kiwi fruit, no need to peel

225g/8oz or ¼ green-fleshed melon, deseeded, peeled, cut into slices that will fit in the juicer chute

25g/1oz/1 cup baby spinach leaves

175g/6oz or 1 small courgette/zucchini

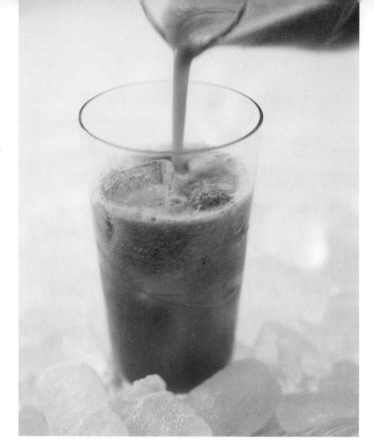

Green goddess

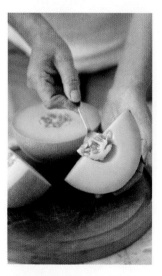

Having a stressful day? Don't reach for the chocolate bar or cookie jar. This delicately sweet and soothing juice is the perfect stressbuster and not only is it lower in calories but it is bursting with vitamins and minerals too.

1 Gradually press all the ingredients through a juicer then pour into a tall glass and serve.

FIGHT THE EFFECTS OF STRESS AND AGING – Just 1 kiwi fruit provides an adult's daily recommended amount of vitamin C or 40mg which is known to not only boost the immune system but also to fight the effects of stress and ageing. Vitamin C also helps to produce the neurotransmitters noradrenaline, which regulates blood flow, and serotonin which is the natural chemical that helps to lift your mood and aid sleep.

Energy 121kcal/509kJ; Protein 5.9g; Carbohydrate 22.3g, of which sugars 21.9g; Fat 1.4g, of which saturates 0.2g; Cholesterol 0mg; Calcium 133mg; Fibre 0.6g; Sodium 93mg.

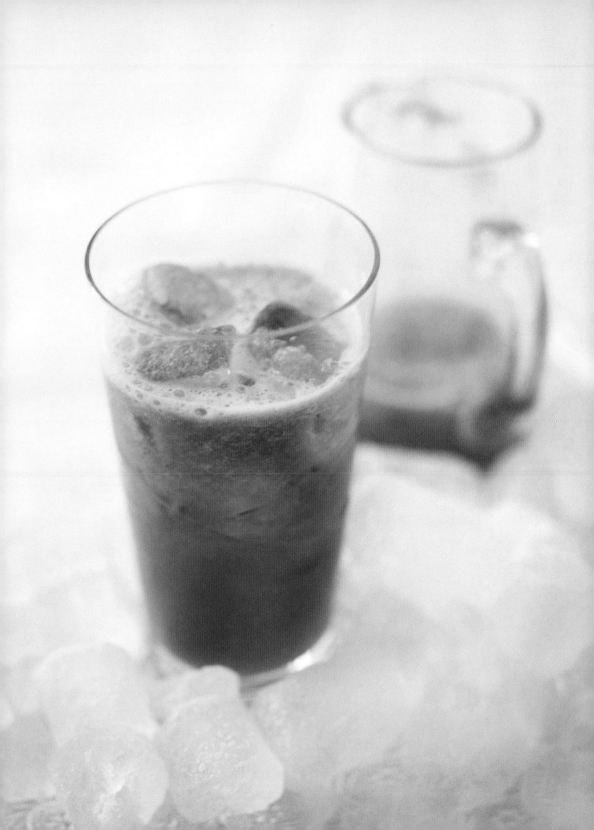

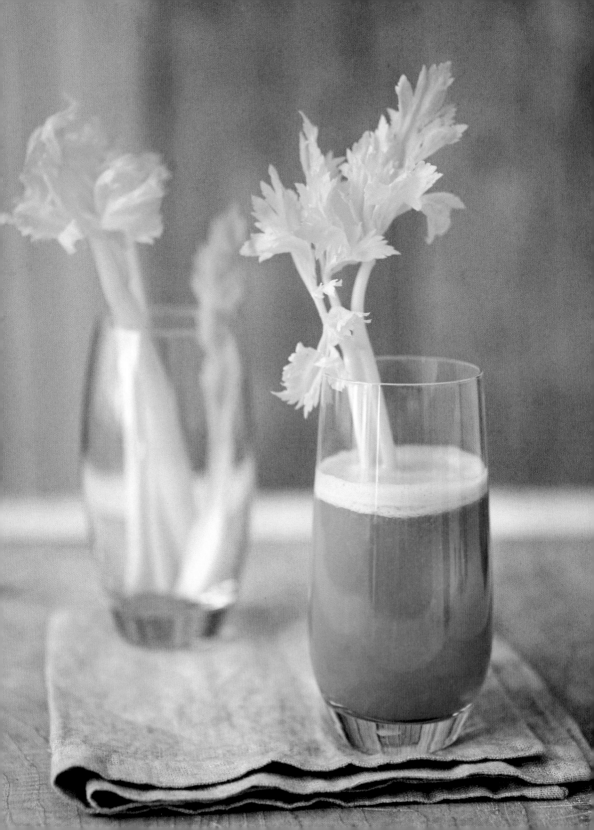

Gingered thirst quencher

The perfect summery cocktail to enjoy with ice, this juice is light, delicate and refreshing with just a hint of ginger. Don't be tempted to be over-generous with the ginger or you will overpower the other flavours.

1 Gradually press all the ingredients through a juicer.

2 Pour into a tall tumbler half-filled with ice cubes and serve with celery stick stirrers, if liked.

LOVE THOSE LEAVES – Low in calories, just one cup of shredded lettuce contains 12 calories. But not all lettuces are the same nutritionally: romaine lettuce has 11% vitamin C, compared to just 1% in iceberg lettuce. Surprisingly just 25g/1oz of romaine lettuce contains 36% of our daily needs of vitamin K, not bad for a vegetable that is practically all water.
AS COOL AS A CUCUMBER – With cucumbers containing 95% water they really are cooling and rehydrating. Plus they contain the mineral silica for good nail health and small amounts of vitamins K, B and C.
COOK'S TIP – As apples vary in size you may need to cut it in half, or even quarters to fit into the chute of your juicer. Make sure to serve this immediately as the apple will oxidize and brown as it stands.

JUICE **SERVES 1**

½ romaine lettuce heart

½ cucumber

1cm/½in slice root ginger, no need to peel

5cm/2in piece broccoli stem

1 stick celery

1 green apple

ice cubes and an extra stick of celery (optional), to serve

Energy 68kcal/282kJ; Protein 3.2g; Carbohydrate 11.8g, of which sugars 11.7g; Fat 1.1g, of which saturates 0.2g; Cholesterol 0mg; Calcium 68mg; Fibre 0.5g; Sodium 26mg.

Summer salad bowl

JUICE **SERVES 1**

15g/½oz/1 cup rocket/
arugula leaves
100g/4oz/generous ½ cup
green seedless grapes
½ romaine lettuce
¼ cucumber
1 stick of celery

All the flavours of a summery salad but in a glass. This super low-calorie drink has slightly peppery undertones with just a hint of celery; if you are a fan of a bloody Mary, you will love this.

1 Gradually press all the ingredients through the juicer. Pour into a tall glass and serve, with lettuce leaf stirrers, if liked.

ROCKET FUEL – While most of us just tend to add rocket or arugula to a mixed leafy salad, it has so much more nutritionally than an average lettuce. Related to kale it contains powerful antioxidants, and is an excellent source of vitamins C and K, plus folates, copper and iron. Some even think it has aphrodisiac properties.

NUTRIENT NOTE – Our brains are made up of 75% water and our muscles about 70% so staying hydrated is vitally important and even more so in hot weather or after exercise.

COOK'S TIP – Celery does have a surprisingly strong taste, even though it is primarily made up of water. If you are not a fan then simply leave it out and replace with a few broccoli florets or half a courgette or zucchini.

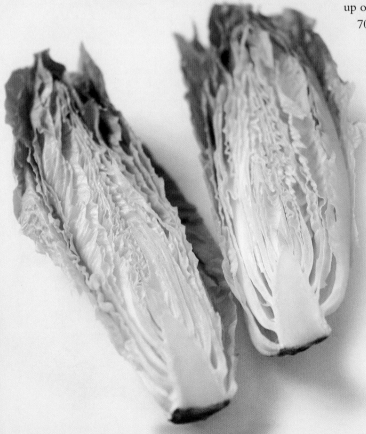

Energy 89kcal/376kJ; Protein 2.5g;
Carbohydrate 18.7g, of which sugars 18.6g; Fat
1g, of which saturates 0.1g; Cholesterol 0mg;
Calcium 85mg; Fibre 0.4g; Sodium 44mg.

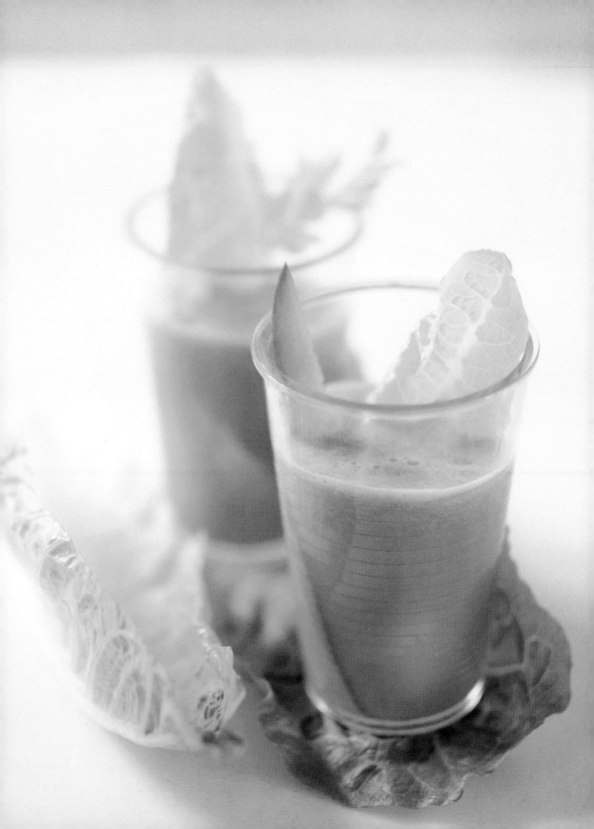

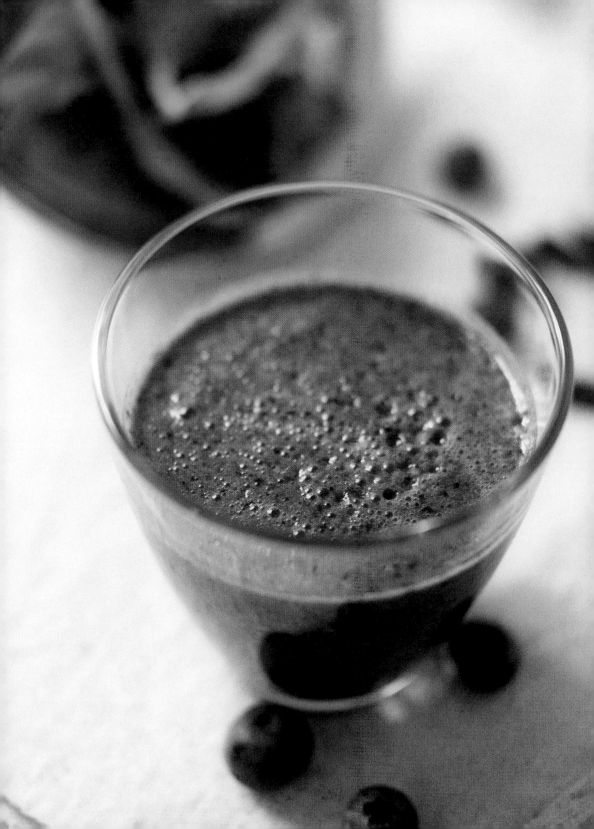

Blueberry booster

This might look like an imposter in a green juice book but it is a good way to get green veg into members of the family who are anti anything green. The fruit completely masks the flavour of the spinach, while protein-boosting goji berries add an extra sweetness.

1 Add all the ingredients to a blender goblet, add the lid and blend until smooth with fine speckles. Pour into a tall glass and serve.

BRILLIANT BLUEBERRIES – Like cranberries, blueberries can be a valuable aid against recurrent urinary tract infections such as cystitis. Researchers are currently seeing if they may also help protect against worsening vision through age-related glaucoma and cataracts, but more information is needed.

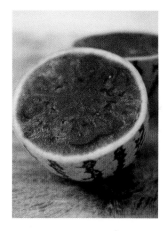

BLEND SERVES 1

75g/3oz/½ cup blueberries

225g/8oz or a 5cm/2in thick wedge of watermelon, peel cut away, flesh cut into chunks

25g/1oz/1 cup baby spinach leaves

½ orange, freshly squeezed juice and the flesh scraped from inside the shell

10ml/2 tsp dried goji berries

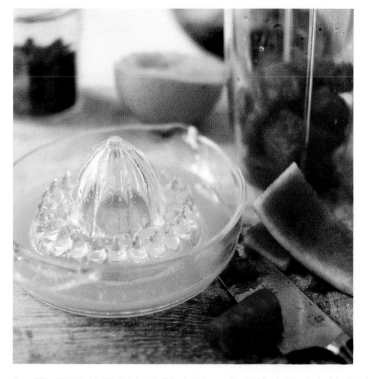

Energy 280kcal/639kJ; Protein 3.9g; Carbohydrate 40.3g, of which sugars 34g; Fat 1.3g, of which saturates 0.3g; Cholesterol 0mg; Calcium 86mg; Fibre 5g; Sodium 43mg.

Broccoli and watercress spritzer

JUICE **SERVES 1**

15g/½oz/1 cup watercress

225g/8oz or ¼ green-fleshed melon, deseeded, peeled, cut into slices that will fit in the juicer shoot

1cm/½in piece root ginger, no need to peel

½ pear, no need to peel or core

75g/3oz broccoli florets and sliced stem

125ml/4fl oz/½ cup sparkling mineral water, chilled

Uber-healthy, low-calorie and alcohol-free and what's more it tastes good too!

1 Press the watercress into the feeder chute of the juicer, then gradually press the melon, ginger, pear and broccoli through the juicer. Pour into a tall glass and top up with sparkling mineral water.

WONDERFUL WATERCRESS – Often overshadowed by trendier rocket/arugula, watercress is high in bone-building and strengthening vitamin K and vitamin A which is important for eye health. It also contains flavonoid antioxidants carotene, lutein and zeaxanthin, which not only support good vision but benefit the cardiovascular system and help protect cells from free radical damage.

NUTRIENT NOTE – The skin reflects what is going on inside the body; if we are stressed or run down our skin will look tired and lifeless. A healthy juice is like giving your body a facial from the inside out.

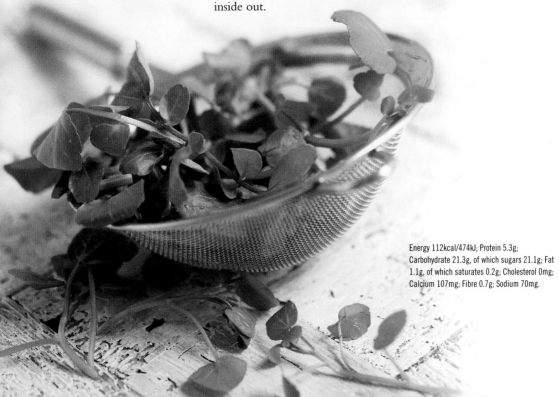

Energy 112kcal/474kJ; Protein 5.3g; Carbohydrate 21.3g, of which sugars 21.1g; Fat 1.1g, of which saturates 0.2g; Cholesterol 0mg; Calcium 107mg; Fibre 0.7g; Sodium 70mg.

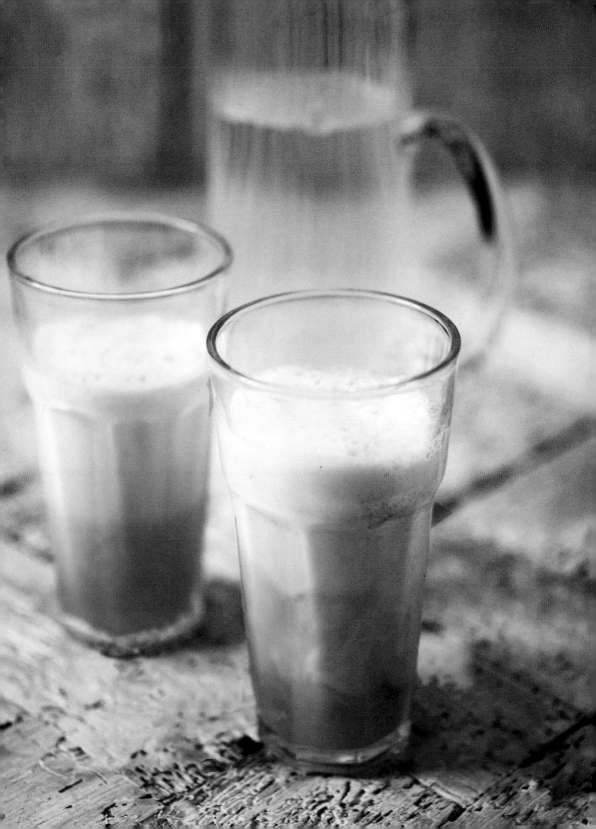

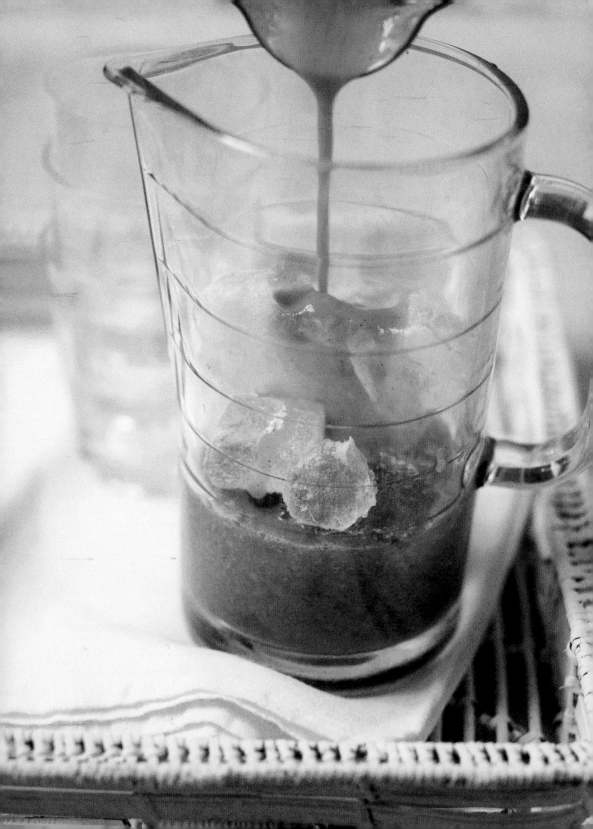

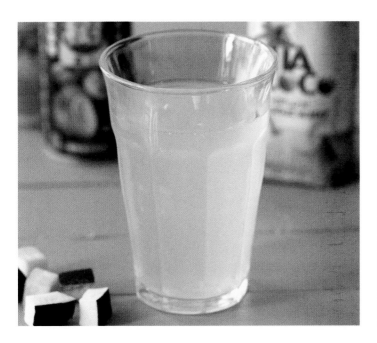

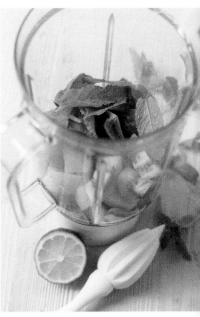

Minted melon crush

This smooth operator is refreshingly cool on a hot day and will quickly rehydrate you and boost vitamin and mineral levels. Forget about Moroccan mint tea, this low-sugar version is much healthier.

1 Add all the ingredients to a blender goblet, add the lid and blitz until smooth. Pour into a tall glass over ice cubes to serve.

SURPRISE SURPRISE – 2 peeled kiwi fruit contain more fibre than a bowl of bran cereal.

NUTRIENT NOTE – There are some big claims out there for the benefits of coconut water from anti-ageing to anti-carcinogenic and anti-thrombotic. While they may not all be true, this clear, slightly nutty-tasting liquid does contain easily digested carbohydrate in the form of sugar plus 5 essential electrolyte minerals, calcium, magnesium, phosphorus, potassium and sodium.

COOK'S TIP – Lacuma is a fruit found growing in Peru; sold in powdered form in the health food store, it is a natural sweetener.

BLEND SERVES 1

200g/7oz or ¼ green-fleshed melon, deseeded, peeled, flesh cut into chunks

1 kiwi fruit, peeled, roughly chopped

6 mint leaves

25g/1oz/1 cup baby spinach leaves

225ml/8fl oz/1 cup coconut water from a carton

juice of ½ lime

5ml/1 tsp lacuma powder

ice cubes, to serve

Energy 90kcal/379kJ; Protein 2.7g; Carbohydrate 19.1g, of which sugars 18.9g; Fat 0.7g, of which saturates 0g; Cholesterol 0mg; Calcium 89mg; Fibre 4.3g; Sodium 91mg.

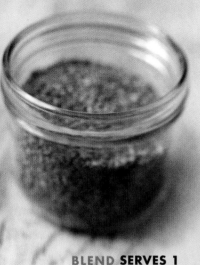

Cacao cup

When dieting you often long for that chocolate fix. This comforting, creamy-tasting smoothie is dairy-free and flavoured with a little raw cacao powder and vanilla for an intense taste that's rich in protein and lower in calories than your usual dairy chocolate drink.

1 Add all the ingredients to a blender goblet, secure the lid and blitz until smooth. Pour into a cup or glass and serve sprinkled with a few extra chia seeds if liked.

NUTRIENT NOTE – Flaxseeds are super-rich in omega 3 fatty acids and fibre, and are one of the richest sources of plant lignans, which are antioxidants and phytoestrogens. They are gluten-free and cholesterol-free too. Always grind the seeds when adding to a shake so that the body can absorb as much of the nutritional content as possible during digestion.

COOK'S TIP – Choose unsweetened almond milk to keep calories as low as possible – or why not make your own, see p19.

BLEND **SERVES 1**

½ banana, sliced

½ pear, cored, leave skin on, cut into chunks

25g/1oz/1 cup baby spinach leaves

10ml/2 tsp cacao powder

10ml/2 tsp ground golden flaxseeds

10ml/2 tsp pea protein or hemp powder

5ml/1 tsp chia seeds

250ml/8fl oz/1 cup unsweetened almond milk

Energy 250kcal/1054kJ; Protein 21.8g; Carbohydrate 26.7g, of which sugars 23.6g; Fat 6.8g, of which saturates 1.6g; Cholesterol 0mg; Calcium 92mg; Fibre 8.4g; Sodium 349mg.

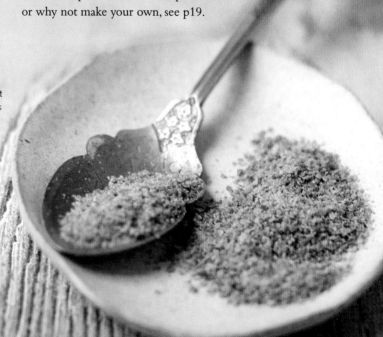

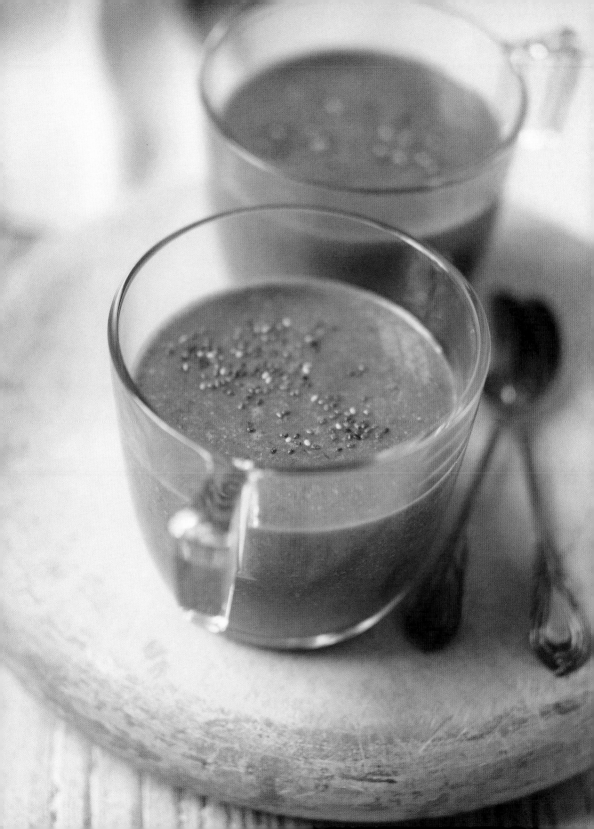

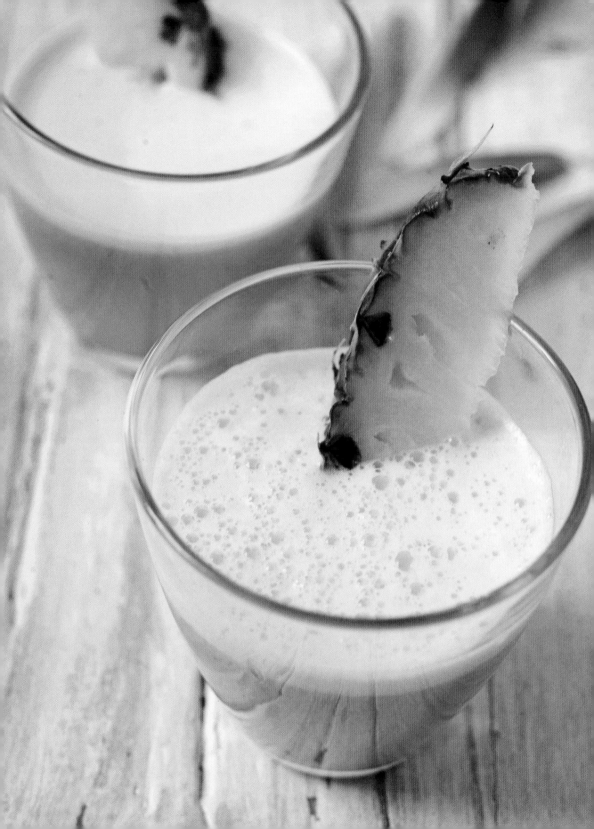

Pineapple pleaser

A light, refreshing frothy juice with just a hint of broccoli. Pineapple is low in calories at just 41 per 100g/3¾oz peeled weight, rich in vitamins A and C, and is a great source of essential minerals, manganese for energy production, potassium to help regulate heart rate and blood pressure, and copper for red blood synthesis.

1 Press the pineapple and all the vegetables through the juicer then pour into a tall glass. Add pineapple slice stirrers, if liked, and serve.

NUTRIENT NOTE – Juicing and smoothie-making is a great way to get you started on a healthier regime and once you begin to cut out the junk foods the less you will crave them.
COOK'S TIP – To get the maximum juice out of your pineapple store it at room temperature before cutting.

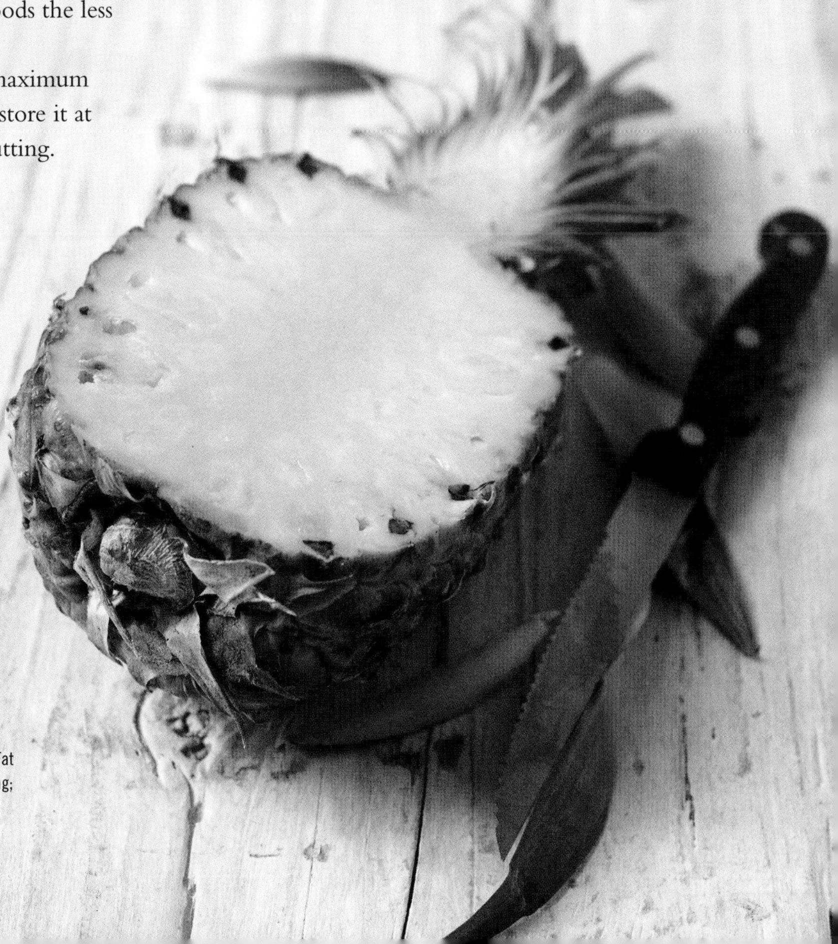

JUICE **SERVES 1**

¼ medium pineapple, skin cut away but core left in, or 200g/7oz/1 cup prepared pineapple, cut into chunks

75g/3oz broccoli florets and sliced stem

100g/4oz courgette/zucchini

100g/4oz cucumber

Energy 135kcal/570kJ; Protein 6.6g; Carbohydrate 24.9g, of which sugars 24.4g; Fat 1.6g, of which saturates 0.2g; Cholesterol 0mg; Calcium 121mg; Fibre 0.7g; Sodium 14mg.

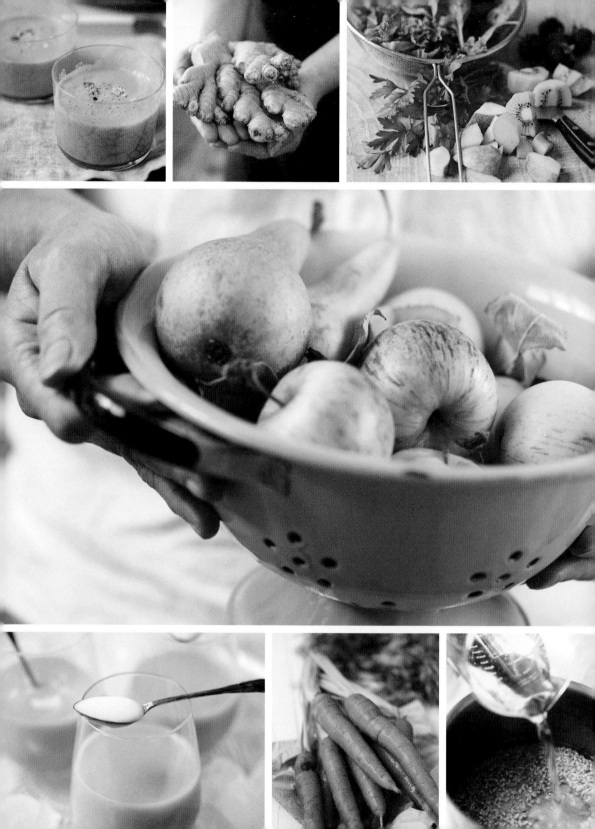

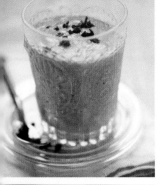

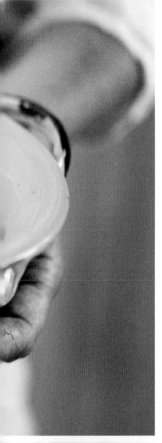

HEALTH SUPER-BOOSTERS

In recent decades the Western world has become overfed, yet undernourished. The life expectancy of our children is dropping, which cannot be right, and our consumption of junk food has increased. Vegetables and fruit act as nature's medicines to keep our bodies in tip-top shape, helping to protect against cancer, cardiovascular disease, strokes, diabetes and obesity. Rich in vitamins and minerals for optimum health, these delicious blends naturally boost our immunity and vitality.

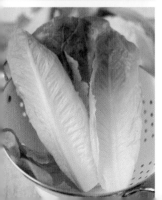

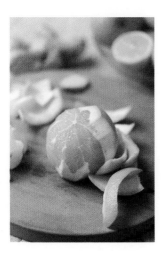

First defence

Fight those winter cold and flu bugs with this foodie fusion, old-fashioned lemon barley water blended with a more modern green spinach-based smoothie.

1 Add the pearl barley and water to a pan, bring to the boil then cover the pan and simmer gently for 30 minutes. Drain the barley through a sieve or strainer and collect the liquid in a measuring jug or cup. You should have about 300ml/ ½ pint/1¼ cups barley water.

2 Add 150ml/¼ pint/⅔ cup of the warm barley water and 30ml/2 tbsp of the cooked barley to a blender goblet then add the orange, lemon, ginger and spinach. Secure the lid and blitz until smooth. Pour into a glass and stir in honey or sweetener of choice, to taste. Serve warm.

BLEND **SERVES 1**

100g/3¾oz/½ cup pearl (pot) barley

600ml/1 pint/2½ cups water

1 orange, zest and pith cut away, cut into chunks

½ lemon, zest and pith cut away, cut into chunks

1 small slice fresh root ginger, no need to peel, quartered

25g/1oz/1 cup baby spinach leaves

5ml/1 tsp honey or sweetener of choice

SUPERHERO CITRUS FRUIT – Fresh lemon juice has long been thought of as a remedy for the common cold. Both lemons and oranges are rich in vitamin C which helps fight infection, aids healing and is needed for healthy teeth and gums, skin, bones and cartilage.

THE IMPORTANCE OF FIBRE – Cooked barley, mixed fruits and vegetables are a great way to boost fibre in blender-style drinks. Increased fibre intakes help to significantly lower the risk of developing coronary heart disease, stroke, hypertension, diabetes, obesity and some gastrointestinal diseases, and it can help lower blood pressure and cholesterol levels and improve insulin sensitivity.

COOK'S TIP – Keep back another 30ml/2 tbsp of cooked barley and the remaining barley water so that you can make this drink again. The remaining cooked barley makes a great high-fibre salad base: mix with chopped herbs, diced tomato, shredded kale, grated carrot and perhaps a little crumbled feta cheese, all tossed in a lemony vinaigrette dressing.

Energy 112kcal/474kJ; Protein 3.3g; Carbohydrate 24.9g, of which sugars 24.9g; Fat 0.6g, of which saturates 0.1g; Cholesterol 0mg; Calcium 187mg; Fibre 3.4g; Sodium 55mg.

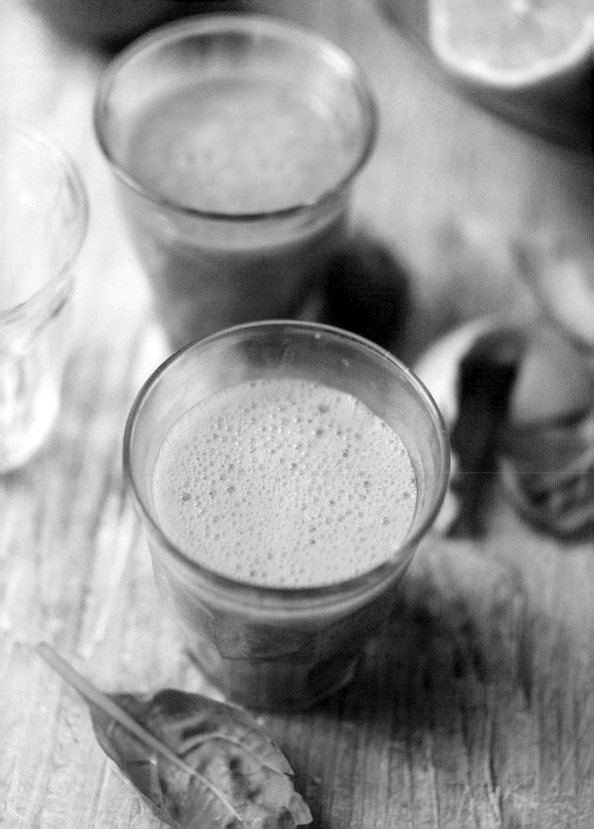

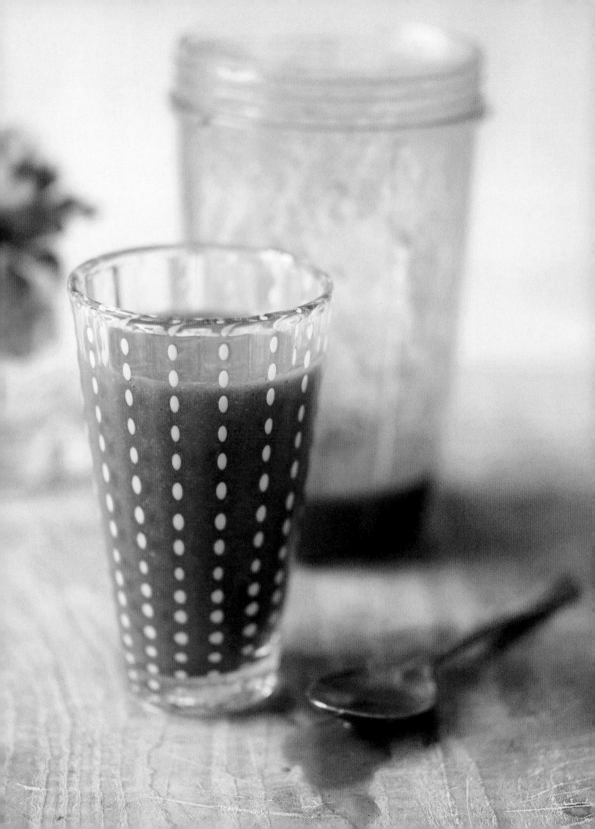

Immune booster

The immune system is essential in protecting our health; each illness, injury or threat to our body stimulates a response for the body to heal itself. Vitamin C is crucial to maintaining and boosting immune levels and as it can't be stored by the body it is needed on a daily basis. This one tasty and refreshing drink is all it takes to keep us on track.

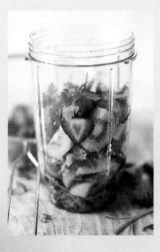

1 Add all the ingredients to a liquidizer goblet, secure the lid and blitz together until smooth. Pour into a tall glass to serve.

COOK'S TIP – Packs of ready-ground flaxseeds are sold in the supermarket and could also be used in place of the homemade ground seed mix.

NUTRIENT NOTE – Diet is important but our lifestyle also plays a significant role too. Smokers need double the amount of vitamin C than non-smokers due to the oxidative stress from the tobacco. Working long hours, feeling constantly stressed and tired can weaken your body's natural immunity so that you become more susceptible to viruses and bacterial infections.

BLEND **SERVES 1**

15g/½oz/½ cup shredded kale

15g/½oz/½ cup baby spinach leaves

10g/¼oz/½ cup parsley

1 kiwi fruit, peeled, cut into chunks

½ pear, cored, skin left on, cut into chunks

50g/2oz/2 strawberries, hulled

15ml/1 tbsp ground seed mix, see p47

125ml/4fl oz/½ cup water

Energy 295kcal/1233kJ; Protein 8.8g; Carbohydrate 44.6g, of which sugars 44.3g; Fat 10g, of which saturates 1.6g; Cholesterol 0mg; Calcium 266mg; Fibre 14g; Sodium 79mg.

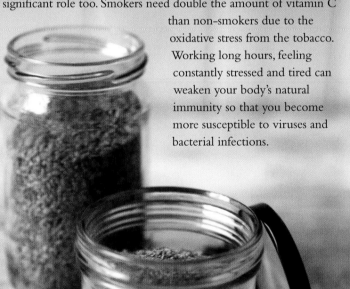

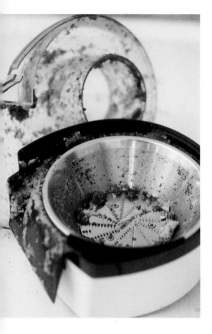
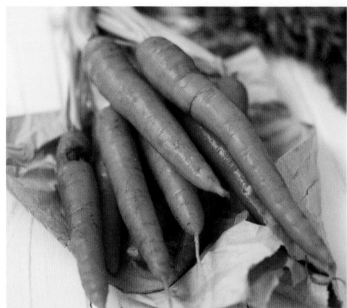

Antioxidant superfusion

JUICE SERVES 1

25g/1oz/1 cup shredded kale

50g/2oz broccoli florets and 5cm/2in piece broccoli stem

2 green apples

150g/5oz or 2 small carrots, scrubbed

50g/2oz or 1 small chunk red cabbage

ice cubes, to serve (optional)

The brighter the colour of the fruit and vegetable, the more antioxidants and phytochemicals there will be. These help to reduce the activity of free radicals in the body which can damage DNA and body tissues, and help to protect against disease. Think of this juice rather like drinking in a rainbow.

1 Gradually press all the vegetables and fruit through the juicer then pour into a tall glass over ice cubes, if liked.

NUTRIENT NOTE – Antioxidants are rather like our bodyguard and are made up of beta-carotene, vitamin C and E, plus the minerals selenium, zinc, copper and manganese, and the carotenoids alpha-carotene, lycopene and lutein. There is growing evidence that antioxidants may help protect against cancer, and reduce the risk of age-related diseases such as Alzheimer's, cataracts, Parkinson's and heart disease.

Energy 154kcal/646kJ; Protein 5.1g; Carbohydrate 31.5g, of which sugars 30.3g; Fat 1.6g, of which saturates 0.3g; Cholesterol 0mg; Calcium 134mg; Fibre 1.2g; Sodium 60mg.

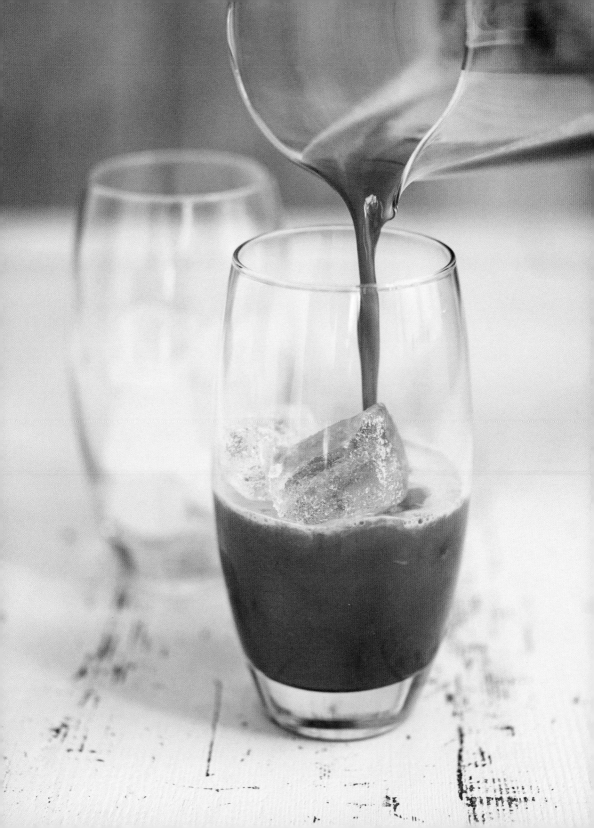

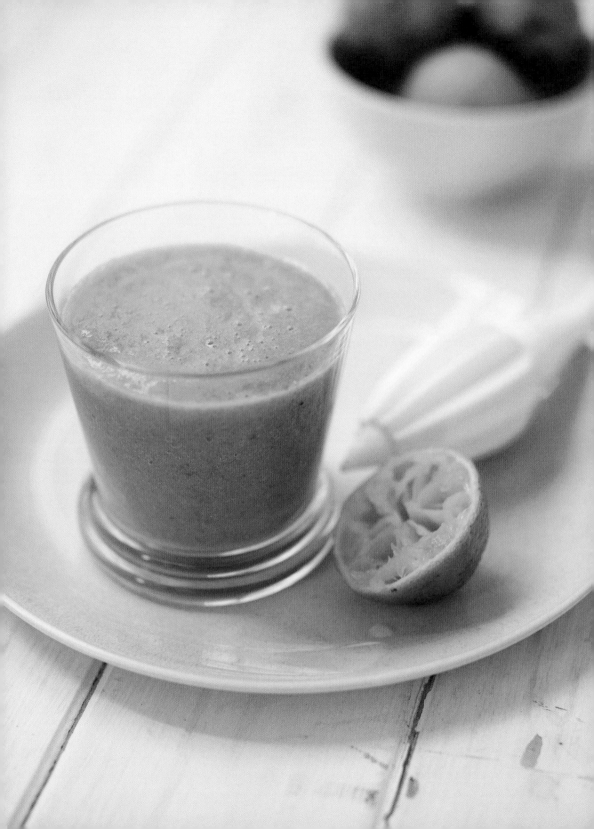

Digestive soother

Our digestive system breaks down the food that we eat into easily absorbed nutrients to build and maintain cells in our body, but it is only as good as the foods that we put in. Just like a car, add the wrong kind or poor-quality fuel and the engine won't perform as well. If you have over-indulged and are suffering with indigestion try this gingered barley and banana smoothie to calm and settle your tummy.

1 Add the cooled barley water to a blender goblet with the ginger, cauliflower and grapes. Add the banana and lettuce then secure the lid and blitz until smooth. Pour into a glass and add lime juice to taste, if liked.

CUT THE GAS – Ginger has a carminative effect and can help to reduce gas and discomfort with indigestion while also easing the feeling of nausea. Easy-to-make barley water also helps to reduce gas and can lessen bloating too.

BLEND SERVES 1

150ml/¼ pint/⅔ cup barley water, see p102

1 thin slice fresh root ginger, no need to peel

50g/2oz/2 cauliflower florets

75g/3oz/½ cup seedless grapes

1 small banana, broken into pieces

4 outer romaine lettuce leaves

fresh lime juice (optional)

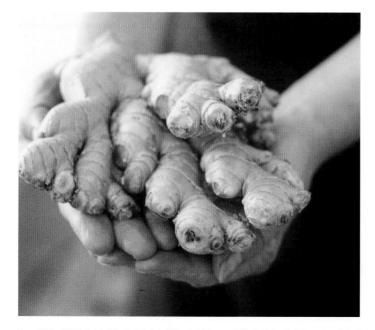

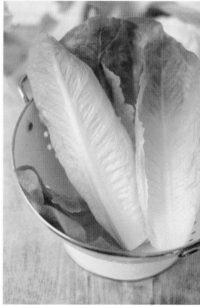

Energy 177kcal/753kJ; Protein 3.8g; Carbohydrate 40.7g, of which sugars 38.7g; Fat 1.1g, of which saturates 0.2g; Cholesterol 0mg; Calcium 40mg; Fibre 4g; Sodium 12mg.

Heartburn healer

BLEND **SERVES 1**

125ml/4fl oz/½ cup plain low-fat or non-dairy yogurt

½ banana, broken into pieces

½ papaya, deseeded, no need to peel, cut into chunks

25g/1oz/1 cauliflower floret

25g/1oz/1 cup baby spinach leaves

10g/¼oz/10 almonds, plus a few extra chopped nuts to decorate, if liked

125ml/4fl oz/½ cup water

If you have over-indulged a little with too much rich food or a glass or two of wine more than you should have had, this soothing yogurt-based smoothie may help to relieve symptoms of heartburn or acid reflux. Papaya contains the natural enzyme 'papain' which is used as an ingredient in many acid reflux medicines.

1 Add all the ingredients to a blender goblet, secure the lid and blitz until smooth. Adjust with a little extra water if preferred then pour into a glass, sprinkle with some extra chopped almonds, if liked, and serve.

YUMMY YOGURT —Yogurt can also help with the bad breath that comes with acid reflux.
HEALTH NOTE — Over-eating not only overloads your digestive system and can lead to acid reflux but so can swallowing too much air. Alcohol and smoking cigarettes can also cause this condition. Seek medical advice if symptoms persist.

Energy 322kcal/1363kJ; Protein 11.9g; Carbohydrate 54.6g, of which sugars 52.5g; Fat 7.7g, of which saturates 1.4g; Cholesterol 2mg; Calcium 340mg; Fibre 11.2g; Sodium 130mg.

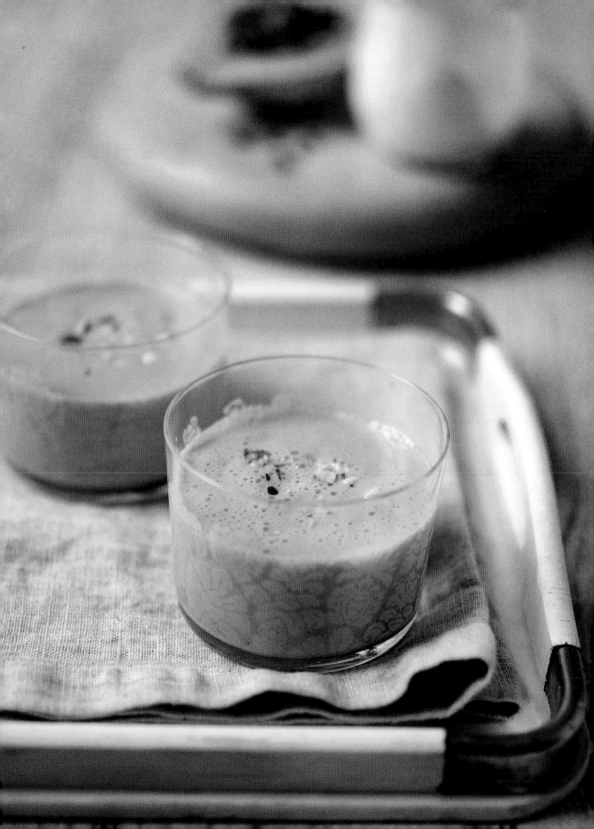

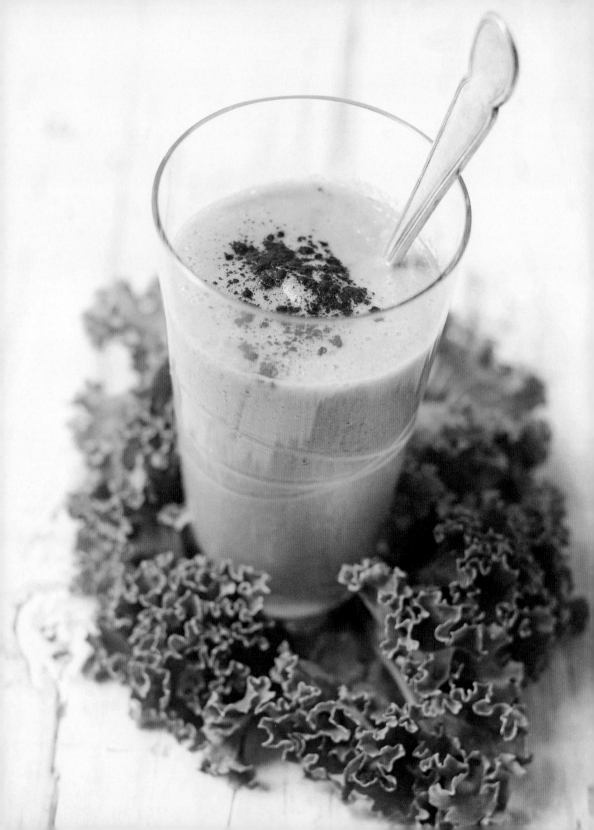

Healthy heart

The World Health Organization says that more people die annually from cardiovascular diseases than from any other cause. By making just small dietary changes, such as introducing a daily juice or shake and maintaining these changes, you can really make a difference to your long-term health.

1 Add all the ingredients to a liquidizer goblet, add the lid and blitz until smooth with just a few green speckles still visible.

2 Pour into a tall glass, sprinkle with spirulina if using, mix with a fork then serve.

LOWERING CHOLESTEROL – High-fibre oats and naturally occurring pectin in pears and apples have been shown to help lower harmful cholesterol and to help regulate blood pressure.
SMALL STEPS MAKE A BIG DIFFERENCE –
Most cardiovascular diseases can be prevented by reducing behavioural risk factors such as tobacco use, unhealthy diet, obesity, physical inactivity and harmful use of alcohol. Stop smoking, cut out the junk food, eat more healthily, drink in moderation and take the stairs rather than the lift or elevator at work, get off the bus one stop early and walk whenever you can.

BLEND SERVES 1

25g/1oz/1 cup shredded kale

25g/1oz/6 sugar snap peas

1 banana, broken into pieces

½ pear, quartered, cored but not peeled, cut into chunks

30ml/2 tbsp rolled oats

250ml/8fl oz/1 cup unsweetened oat milk

1.5ml/¼ tsp spirulina powder (optional)

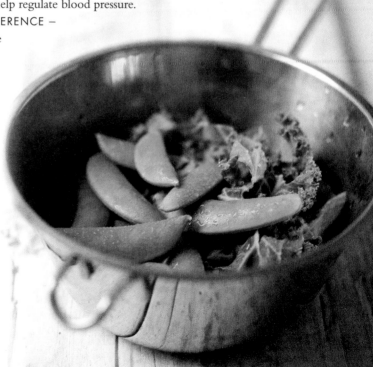

Energy 400kcal/1686kJ; Protein 7.3g; Carbohydrate 56.6g, of which sugars 39.7g; Fat 6.4g, of which saturates 0.2g; Cholesterol 0mg; Calcium 77mg; Fibre 7.9g; Sodium 25mg.

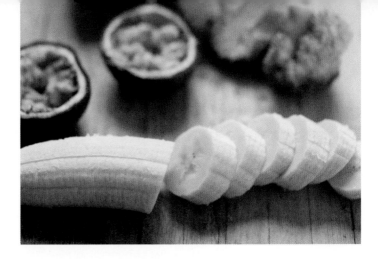

Hormone balance – women

BLEND **SERVES 1**

1 passion fruit, halved

1 small banana, broken into pieces

40g/1½oz/2 broccoli florets

15g/½oz/½ cup shredded kale leaves

15ml/1 tbsp ground seed mix, see p47

15ml/1 tbsp goji berries, plus a few extra to decorate if liked

15ml/1 tbsp dried mixed sea salad

125ml/4fl oz/½ cup plain low-fat or non-dairy yogurt

175ml/6fl oz/¾ cup coconut water from a carton

If you battle with mood swings and poor concentration with PMS and the menopause it can be helpful to include vitamin B and mineral-rich foods in your diet.

1 Scoop the passion fruit seeds into the blender goblet then add the banana, broccoli and kale. Add the ground seed mix, goji berries and sea salad then pour in the yogurt and coconut water.

2 Add the lid and blitz until smooth with fine red speckles. Adjust the thickness with a little water if needed.

3 Pour into a tall glass and serve topped with a few extra chopped goji berries, if liked.

HEALTH NOTE – Some studies suggest that the caffeine from too many cups of coffee and tea can exacerbate PMS. Change to decaf versions or cut down on coffee and tea consumption gradually. MINERAL MAGIC – The body needs 16 essential minerals to function properly. The most important for women are: calcium needed for bones, nerves and muscles, especially important for menopausal women; iron for healthy red blood cells and to help fight fatigue; magnesium for energy release and to aid dopamine production and help the body process oestrogen; potassium to maintain fluid and electrolyte balance; selenium for healthy hair and nails; and finally zinc for efficient functioning of the immune system.

Energy 460kcal/1121kJ; Protein 14.7g; Carbohydrate 42.7g, of which sugars 33.9g; Fat 9.4g, of which saturates 2g; Cholesterol 2mg; Calcium 267mg; Fibre 5.4g; Sodium 92mg.

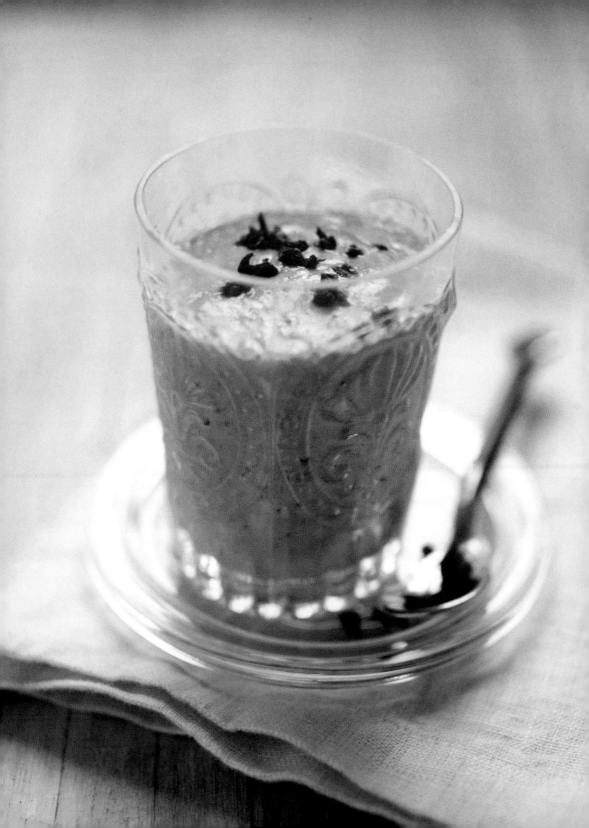

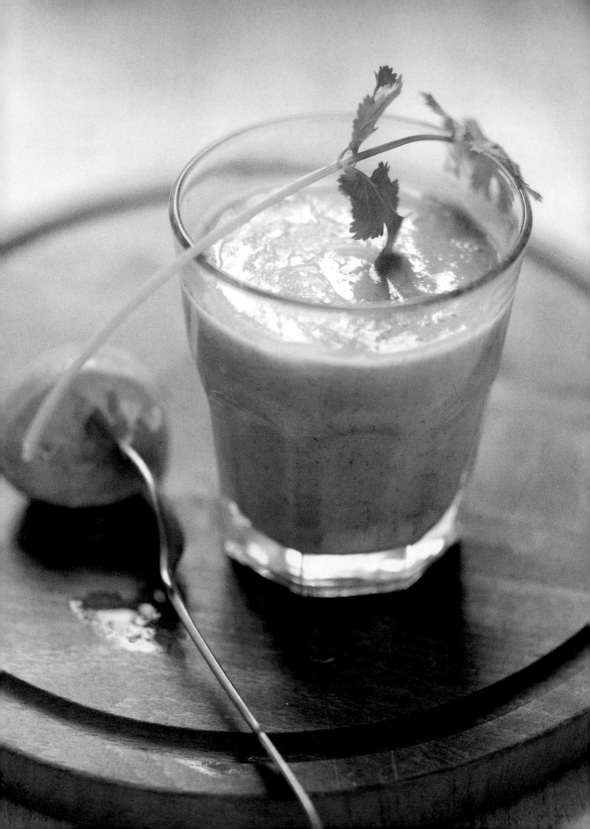

Hormone balance – men

Boost testosterone levels and raise your sex drive with this Mexican-inspired guacamole-style shake.

1 Add the tomato, chilli, kiwi and avocado to the blender goblet then add the kale, ground seeds, almonds and coconut water. Secure the lid and blitz until smooth.

2 Pour into a glass, stir in chopped coriander, and add lime juice to taste.

NUTRIENT NOTE – Dark green leafy vegetables such as kale, spinach and chard are a good source of B vitamins while the ground seeds contain zinc; both are known to boost testosterone levels. Lycopene, the carotenoid pigment that turns tomatoes red, is absorbed more readily by the body when eaten with avocado or avocado oil and may help protect against prostate cancer.
COOK'S TIP – This is quite a thick shake, so stir in a little extra water to get the consistency you prefer.

BLEND **SERVES 1**

1 tomato, cut into quarters

1 slice red chilli

1 kiwi fruit, peeled, cut into chunks

½ small avocado, stoned/pitted, flesh scooped from skin

15g/½oz/½ cup shredded kale

15ml/1 tbsp ground mixed seeds, see p47

10g/¼oz/10 almonds

250ml/8fl oz/1 cup coconut water from a carton, or water

2–3 stems fresh coriander/cilantro, finely chopped

lime juice, to taste

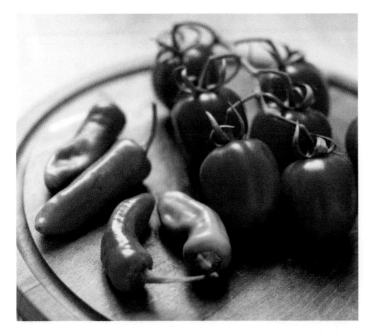

Energy 290kcal/1207kJ; Protein 7.7g; Carbohydrate 13.3g, of which sugars 9.6g; Fat 23.2g, of which saturates 3.6g; Cholesterol 0mg; Calcium 86mg; Fibre 6.6g; Sodium 20mg.

Bone builder

JUICE **SERVES 1**

15g/½oz/1 cup watercress

25g/1oz/1 cup shredded kale

75g/3oz/½ cup broccoli
florets and stem

1 pear, unpeeled and cored

1 orange, zest and
pith cut away

90ml/6 tbsp plain low-fat or
non-dairy yogurt

Your skeleton doesn't actually stop growing until you
are 21. Dairy foods, fortified milks and green leafy
vegetables all help maintain bone strength and health.
Whatever your age, regular exercise as well as a healthy
diet is important to maintain and improve bone strength,
muscle tone and importantly for seniors, balance.

1 Press the watercress and kale through the juicer then add
the broccoli, pear and orange.

2 Pour the juice into a glass and spoon in the yogurt. Stir
lightly for a marbled effect then serve.

NUTRIENT NOTE – Vitamin D aids the absorption
of bone-building calcium, and can be produced
by the action of the sunlight on our body; the
amount depends on how strong the
sunlight is and if you are in
direct sunshine or in the
shade, just 10–20 minutes
outside a day is all it takes.
Vitamin D is also fortified or
added to non-dairy milks.
COOK'S TIP – If you are
avoiding dairy products then
stir natural or plain soya
yogurt into the juice instead.

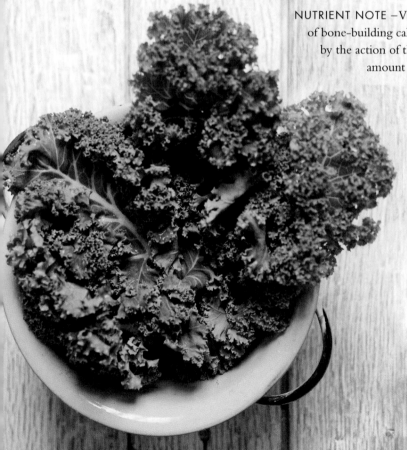

Energy 191kcal/811kJ; Protein 10.7g;
Carbohydrate 33.7g, of which sugars 33.5g; Fat
2.4g, of which saturates 0.8g; Cholesterol 1mg;
Calcium 319mg; Fibre 1.1g; Sodium 91mg.

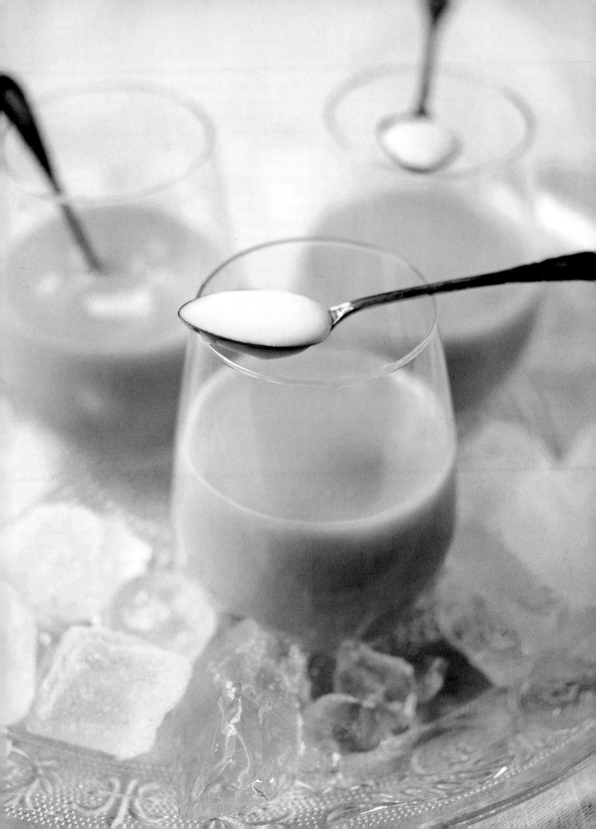

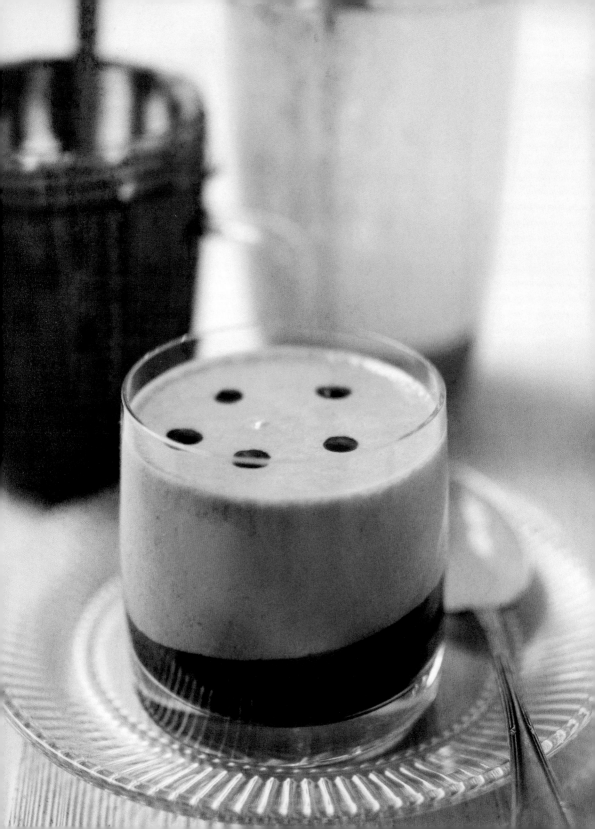

Age defier

This anti-ageing two-tone smoothie is just bursting with antioxidants and good omega 3 fatty acids, that are not only anti-inflammatory but linked to improved brain function, as well as protein, vitamins and minerals to help keep your body at optimum health so that you can live life to the full for longer.

1 Add the blackberries, strawberries and 15ml/1 tbsp of the almond milk to the blender goblet and blitz until smooth. Pour into the base of a glass, reserving 5ml/1 tsp, and set aside.

2 Rinse the blender goblet then add the remaining almond milk, banana, spinach, sea salad, goji berries, flaxseeds and hemp oil. Add the lid and blitz until smooth. Slowly pour the green smoothie into the glass over the back of a teaspoon so that one colour sits on top of the other. Spoon dots of the remaining fruit purée over the top of the smoothie and serve.

NUTRIENT NOTE – As you age you need to maintain protein levels. Every cell in the body needs protein for growth, maintenance and repair and to prevent muscles losing strength.
COOK'S TIP – Sea salad is sold dried and in small shreds and is a mix of dulce, nori and sea lettuce. Look out for packs of Cornish sea salad or if you can't find that in the shops use shredded dulce from Spain. No need to rehydrate before use as it is being mixed with almond milk.

Energy 501kcal/1280kJ; Protein 8.9g; Carbohydrate 43.9g, of which sugars 35.3g; Fat 16g, of which saturates 2g; Cholesterol 0mg; Calcium 103mg; Fibre 7.2g; Sodium 207mg.

BLEND SERVES 1

75g/3oz/generous ¼ cup blackberries

50g/2oz/3 strawberries, hulled

250ml/8floz/1 cup unsweetened almond milk

1 small banana, broken into pieces

25g/1oz/1 cup baby spinach leaves

15ml/1 tbsp dried sea salad

15ml/1 tbsp goji berries

10ml/2 tsp ground flaxseeds

5ml/1 tsp hemp oil

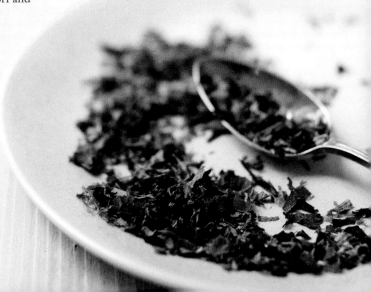

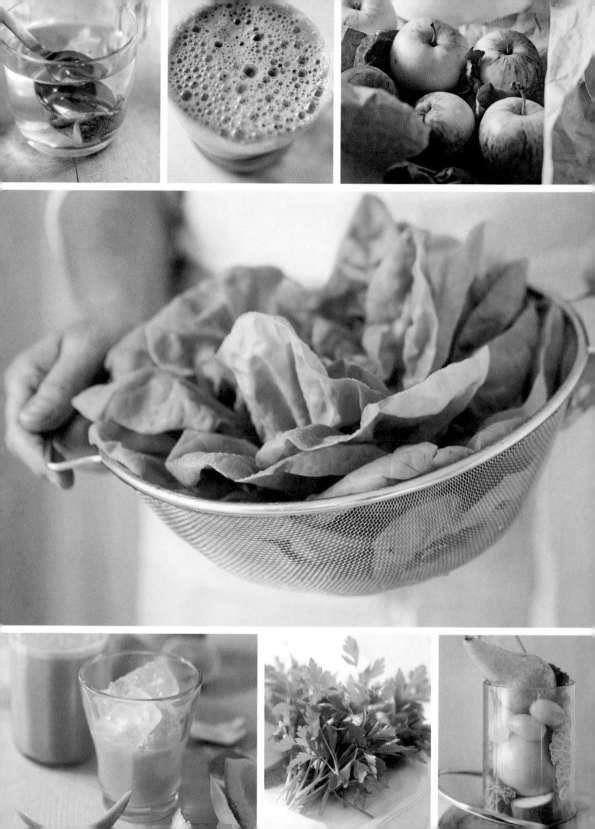

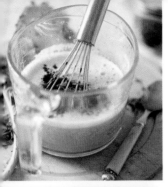

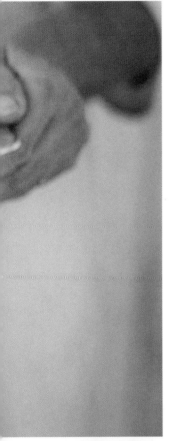

GREEN DETOX

A detox diet is a great time to take a fresh look at what you eat. If you have been over-indulging over Christmas, drinking too much, working too hard or just generally not looking after your body, then a detox for a few days or couple of weeks can be a great way of taking stock. Cut out the junk food, sugary cakes and cookies and introduce a nutrient-packed digestive-soothing juice once or even twice a day. Eat lighter and cleaner, cut out red meat, dairy and wheat, and eat more fibre-rich foods and good fats. Catch up on sleep to reboot and feel better.

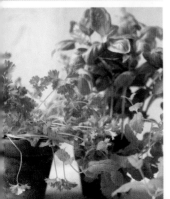

Red cabbage and kale digestive aid

JUICE **SERVES 1**

25g/1oz/1 cup shredded or whole kale leaves

175g/6oz or 1 courgette/zucchini

150g/5oz or 1 carrot, scrubbed

75g/3oz or 1 small parsnip, scrubbed

75g/3oz/scant 1 cup roughly chopped red cabbage

1 stick celery

1 green apple

2.5ml/½ tsp wheatgrass powder

Energy 190kcal/796kJ; Protein 7.5g; Carbohydrate 35.7g, of which sugars 29.3g; Fat 2.7g, of which saturates 0.5g; Cholesterol 0mg; Calcium 204mg; Fibre 1.7g; Sodium 84mg.

A rainbow of colour, don't stir this juice until you are just about to serve. Packed with pure concentrated goodness, it is full of vitamins, minerals, phytochemicals and antioxidants to help fight infection, give strength to muscles, skin, bone and other tissues, and boost production of white blood cells to kick-start your healthy-eating detox.

1 Press the kale into the feeder chute of the juicer, then gradually press all the remaining ingredients except the wheatgrass through.

2 Whisk in the wheatgrass powder, pour into a tall glass and serve.

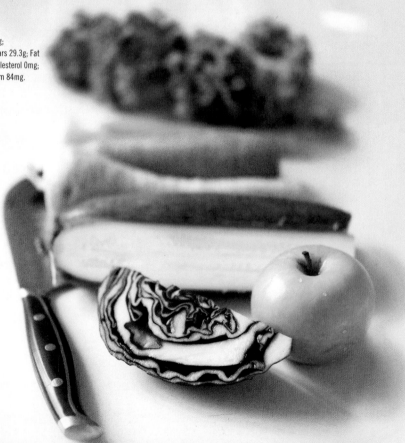

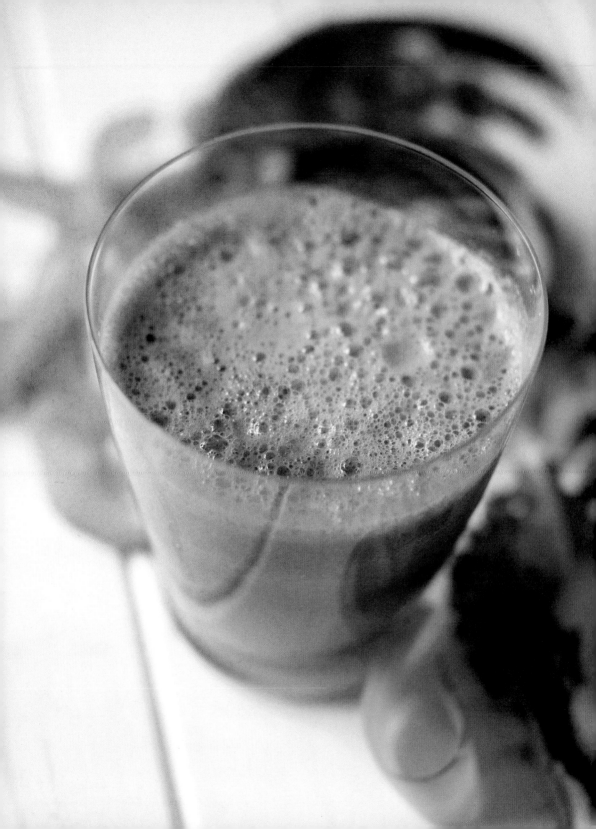

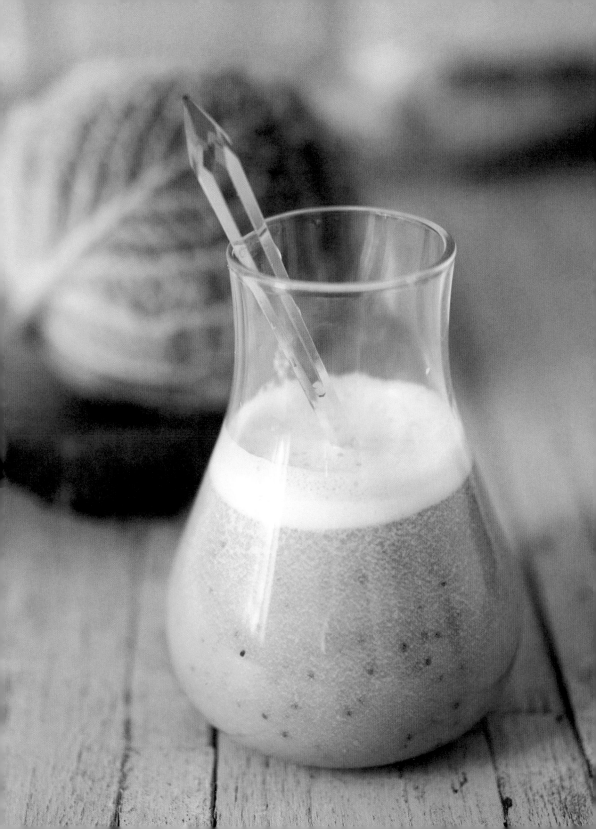

Gorgeous green pep-up

A super-vitality juice with plenty of essential nutrients and natural fruit pectin to help cleanse and soothe the digestive system.

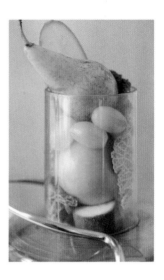

1 Roll the cabbage leaves up and feed through the chute of the juicer then add the courgette, grapes, pear and apple.

2 Pour the juice into a tall glass, stir in the chia seeds and serve immediately.

GORGEOUSLY GREEN – Cabbage might not be top of the list of ingredients to juice but this much maligned vegetable is rich in beta-carotene, vitamins C, E and K plus potassium, not to mention the amino acid glutamine, an anti-inflammatory. Mixed with naturally sweet and soothing fruits its flavour is pretty well disguised. COOK'S TIP – Homemade pear and apple juice quickly turns brown as it stands so make sure to serve this juice the minute that it is made.

JUICE **SERVES 1**

75g/3oz or 2 dark outer green Savoy cabbage leaves

175g/6oz/ 1 courgette/zucchini

100g/3¾oz/generous ½ cup green seedless grapes

1 pear

1 green apple

5ml/1 tsp chia seeds

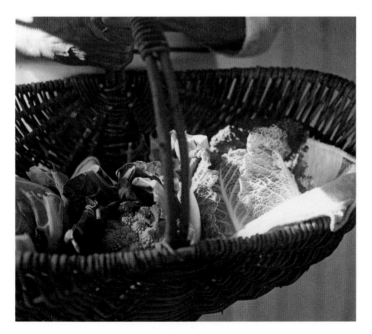

Energy 226kcal/952kJ; Protein 6.9g; Carbohydrate 44.6g, of which sugars 44.2g; Fat 3.1g, of which saturates 0.5g; Cholesterol 0mg; Calcium 141mg; Fibre 1.4g; Sodium 64mg.

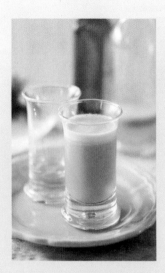

Parslied purifier

Parsley has long been used in herbal medicine as a blood tonic and purifier, natural diuretic and as a digestive aid, and it may even help with bad breath.

1 Press the parsley through the juicer, followed gradually by the spinach, celery and apples. Pour into a glass and stir in the hemp oil.

NUTRIENT NOTE – Hemp seeds contain over 46% oil and this oil is rich in essential fatty acids omega 6 and omega 3; hemp is one of the few plants that contains these fatty acids, making it a great supplement for those on a vegetarian or vegan diet. Plus, it contains all the amino acids, not just the essential ones, and is a good source of tocopherols or vitamin E. Store in the refrigerator.

COOK'S TIP – You don't get a lot of juice from parsley but what you do is a very deep green and adds a unique and delicate flavour.

JUICE **SERVES 1**

15g/½oz/¾ cup fresh parsley

25g/1oz/1 cup baby spinach leaves

1 stick celery

2 green apples

5ml/1 tsp hemp oil

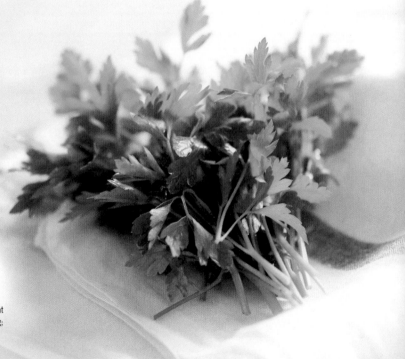

Energy 111kcal/465kJ; Protein 1.9g; Carbohydrate 18.8g, of which sugars 18.7g; Fat 3.6g, of which saturates 0.5g; Cholesterol 0mg; Calcium 91mg; Fibre 0.7g; Sodium 63mg.

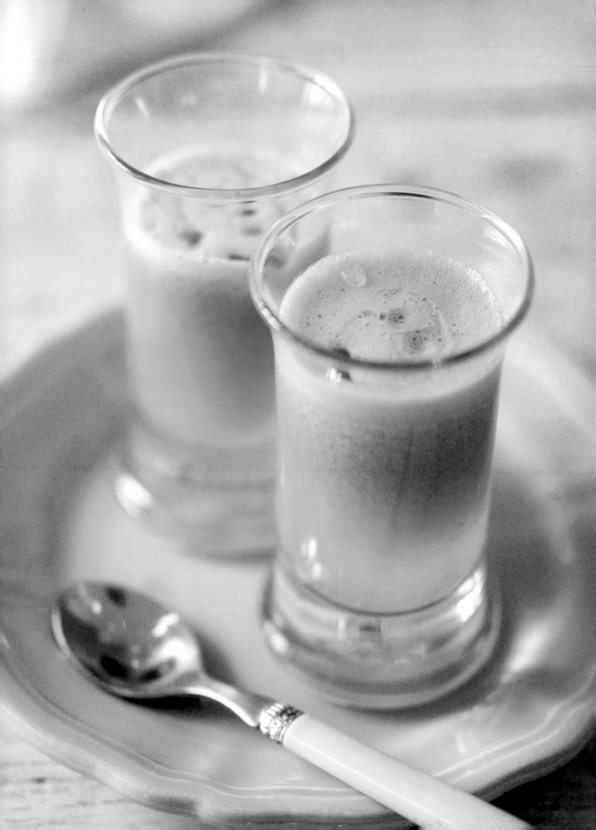

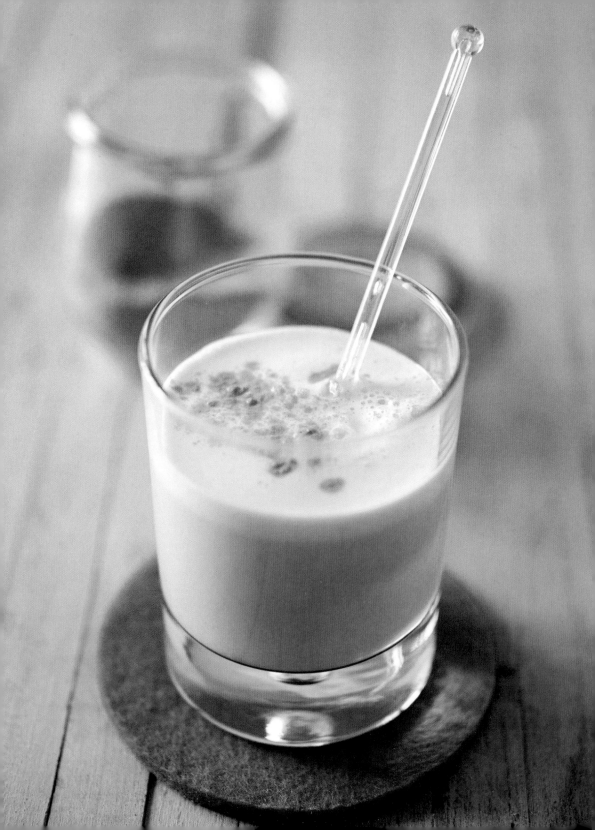

Creamy apple and parsnip soother

Soothe and calm your digestive system and boost
immunity to help fight those winter cold germs.

1 Press all the ingredients through a juicer except the
turmeric then pour into a glass. Stir in the turmeric
and serve.

JUST A PINCH – Long used in natural medicine in China and
India, turmeric is a natural antiseptic and anti-bacterial agent. Fresh
turmeric root is now more widely available in supermarkets and
Indian supermarkets – cut a slice and add to the juicer in much the
same way as root ginger.

NUTRIENT NOTE – Romanesco cauliflowers look
a little like a space-age vegetable with their
knobbly florets. Just like their white
counterparts, the cauliflower contains
vitamin C plus sulphurous compounds
which may help to protect against
various cancers.

COOK'S TIP – Parsnips are at their
sweetest a few weeks after the first frost of
winter as the cold causes the starch they
contain to turn to sugar.

JUICE SERVES 1

2 green apples

75g/3oz or 1 small parsnip,
scrubbed

25g/1oz/1 cup baby
spinach leaves

75g/3oz or 3 florets cut from
a green Romanesco
cauliflower

pinch ground turmeric

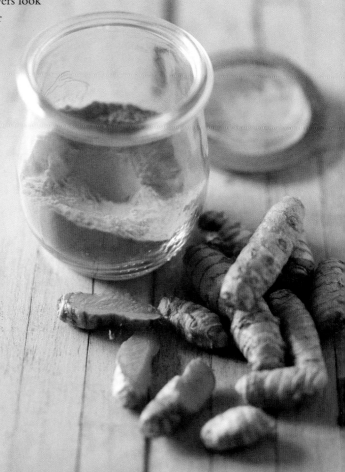

Energy 150kcal/634kJ; Protein 5.4g;
Carbohydrate 29.7g, of which sugars 24.2g; Fat
1.8g, of which saturates 0.3g; Cholesterol 0mg;
Calcium 95mg; Fibre 0.5g; Sodium 54mg.

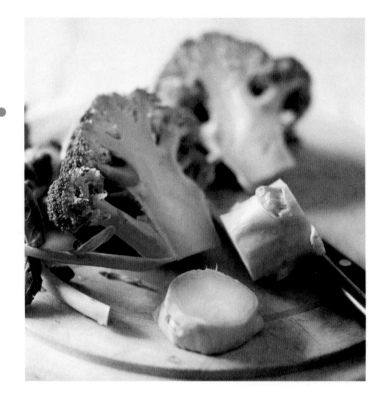

JUICE **SERVES 1**

100g/3¾oz/1 cup broccoli florets and sliced stem

250g/9oz or 1 medium courgette/zucchini

1 green apple

1cm/½in piece fresh root ginger, no need to peel

2.5ml/½ tsp powdered spirulina (optional)

Broccoli body balancer

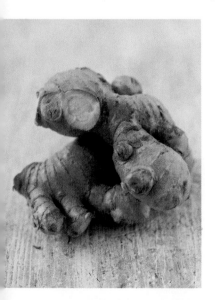

When on a detox, cutting out tea and coffee can be really hard. This refreshing juice makes a much healthier caffeine-free alternative and if you serve it with the spirulina stirred in you will be adding a protein power-boost too.

1 Press the vegetables, apple and ginger through the juicer. Whisk the spirulina into the juice if using, then pour into a tall glass and serve.

SUPERHERO BROCCOLI – Often regarded as one of the top superfoods, broccoli belongs to the cruciferous family along with cauliflower and cabbage. It is a powerful antioxidant, and has high levels of calcium and vitamin K important for bone health and prevention of osteoporosis. The darker the florets the more beta-carotene and vitamin C they contain.

Energy 109kcal/456kJ; Protein 9.2g; Carbohydrate 14.2g, of which sugars 13.7g; Fat 2g, of which saturates 0.5g; Cholesterol 0mg; Calcium 121mg; Fibre 0.8g; Sodium 13mg.

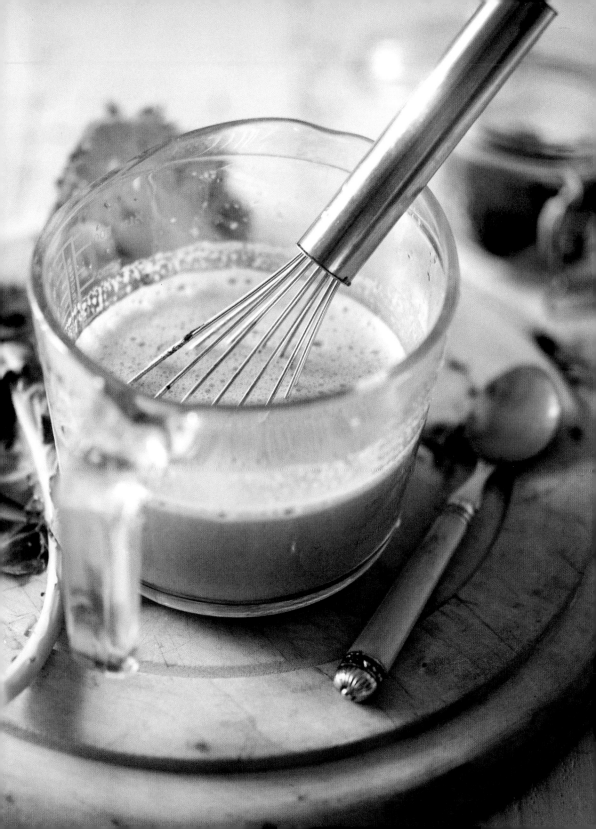

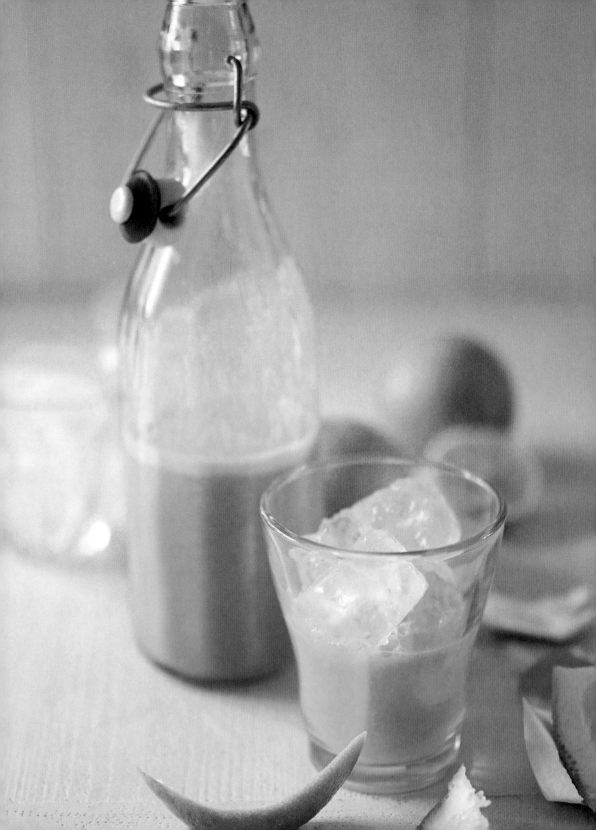

Citrus super-cleanse

Reawaken those tastebuds with this fresh-tasting immune-boosting citrus juice. Grapefruit can be a little sharp but by mixing with orange and pear you have all the zingy freshness balanced with a little soothing and naturally sweet pear juice.

1 Press the kale into the juicer feeder chute then gradually press all the other ingredients through the juicer. Pour into a glass half-filled with ice cubes and serve.

CITRUS FRUITS – This is packed with vitamin C which not only helps fight off infection but also helps with wound-healing, the absorption of iron, and as an antioxidant to help protect against cancer, heart disease and circulatory diseases.
COOK'S TIP – Cut the zest and most of the pith off citrus fruit before you juice or blend. The coloured zest is just too strong-tasting and the pith can be bitter.

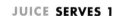

JUICE SERVES 1

25g/1oz/1 cup shredded kale

25g/1oz/1 cup baby spinach leaves

1 grapefruit, rind and pith cut away

1 orange, rind and pith cut away

½ pear, no need to peel or core

ice cubes, to serve

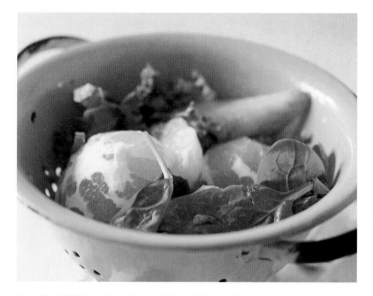

Energy 137kcal/579kJ; Protein 4.4g; Carbohydrate 29.3g, of which sugars 29.3g; Fat 1g, of which saturates 0.1g; Cholesterol 0mg; Calcium 176mg; Fibre 0.3g; Sodium 59mg.

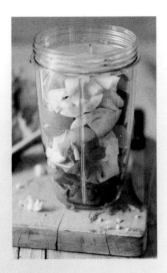

Spring clean

While we all know we should eat at least 5 portions of fruit and veg a day it is easy to get into bad habits. Get back on track with this mild green juice, the gentle way to soothe and cleanse the digestive system.

1 Add all the ingredients to a liquidizer goblet, secure the lid and blitz until smooth. Pour into a tall glass to serve.

NUTRIENT NOTE – Herbalists have long thought of fennel as a help with digestion problems including heartburn, intestinal gas, bloating and loss of appetite. This Mediterranean vegetable has a delicate, slightly sweet anise-like flavour.

BLEND **SERVES 1**

¼ small fennel bulb or ¼ cup when roughly chopped

25g/1oz/1 cup baby spinach leaves

40g/1½oz or 3 small cauliflower florets

½ pear, no need to peel or core, cut into chunks

75g/3oz/½ cup green seedless grapes

250ml/8fl oz/1 cup water

Energy 96kcal/407kJ; Protein 2.8g; Carbohydrate 20.8g, of which sugars 20.6g; Fat 0.7g, of which saturates 0.1g; Cholesterol 0mg; Calcium 71mg; Fibre 0.8g; Sodium 43mg.

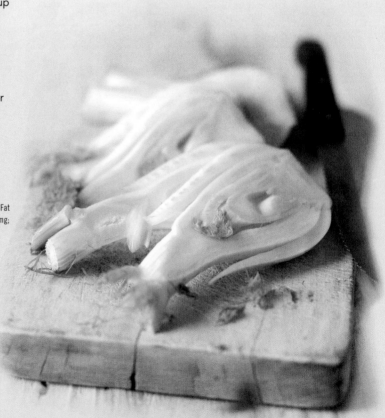

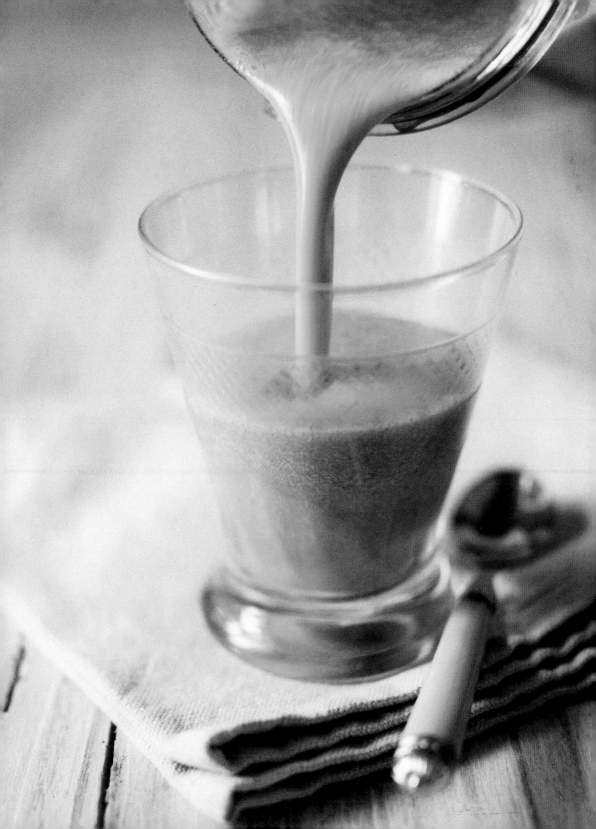

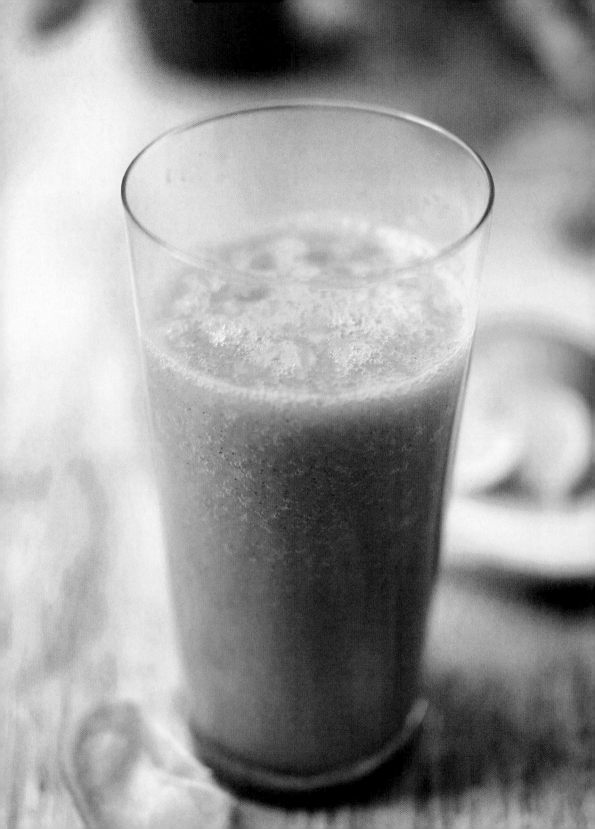

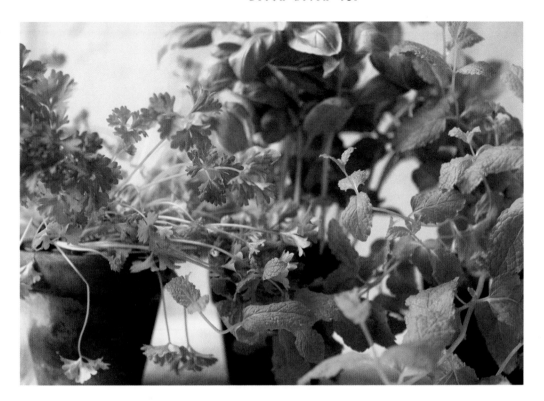

Summer herb sensation

Packed with light flavours, fresh herbs are antibacterial, anti-inflammatory, rich in antioxidants, and taste delicious mixed with refreshing melon and tangy kiwi fruit.

1 Add all the ingredients to the blender goblet except the lime juice and blitz until smooth.

2 Pour into a tall glass and stir in lime juice to taste.

NUTRIENT FACT – Just 15ml/1 tbsp of chopped parsley contains 61.5 micrograms of vitamin K or 77% of the recommended daily allowance.
COOK'S TIP – Transplant pots of supermarket herbs into larger pots at home and keep them on the windowsill or by the back door; water them regularly and they will continue to grow for several months.

BLEND SERVES 1

2 stems fresh parsley
2 stems fresh mint
2 stems fresh basil
¼ green-fleshed melon, deseeded, peeled, cut into chunks
1 kiwi fruit, peeled, cut into chunks
250ml/8fl oz/1 cup water
squeeze of fresh lime, to taste

Energy 70kcal/298kJ; Protein 1.9g; Carbohydrate 15.2g, of which sugars 14.9g; Fat 0.6g, of which saturates 0g; Cholesterol 0mg; Calcium 64mg; Fibre 3.3g; Sodium 54mg.

Chamomile, pear and mint pacifier

BLEND **SERVES 1**

1 chamomile teabag

250ml/8fl oz/1 cup boiling water

8 fresh mint leaves

¼ green-fleshed melon, deseeded, peeled, cut into chunks

handful round/butterhead lettuce leaves, torn into pieces

For many of us going on a detox diet is a way of giving our digestive system a holiday, a time to relax and unwind away from the stresses of a diet loaded with caffeine, alcohol, fat, refined sugar and white flours. This soothing herb tea-based smoothie is the perfect antidote to modern living.

1 Add the teabag to a cup, pour over the boiling water and leave to infuse for 2 minutes then remove the teabag and leave the tea to go cold.

2 Pour the cooled chamomile tea into a blender goblet, add the mint leaves, melon and lettuce leaves. Press on the lid and blitz until smooth. Pour into a tall glass and serve.

LOVE THOSE LEAVES – Lettuce is made up mainly of water which is essential to keep our body hydrated but it does contain the compound lactucarium, which is thought to calm and soothe the nerves and aid sleep. Choose the darker outer green lettuce leaves as these contain the most beta-carotene, vitamin C, folate and iron.

COOK'S TIP – Chamomile flowers have long been made into tea for their fragrant, soothing and calming properties. A teabag is the easiest way of making up this tea, but if you would rather use loose tea leaves use 2.5ml/½ tsp.

Energy 78kcal/330kJ; Protein 3.1g; Carbohydrate 13.5g, of which sugars 13.5g; Fat 1.6g, of which saturates 0.3g; Cholesterol 0mg; Calcium 104mg; Fibre 4.4g; Sodium 56mg.

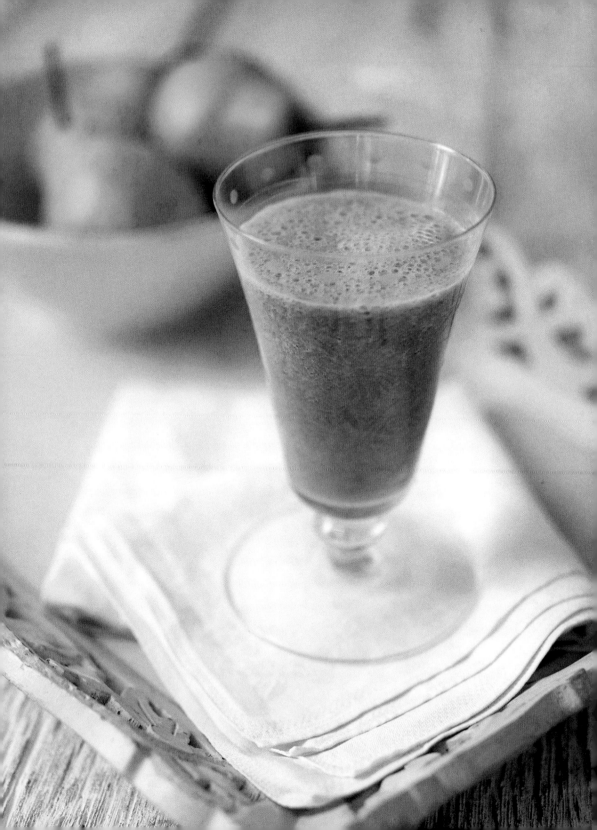

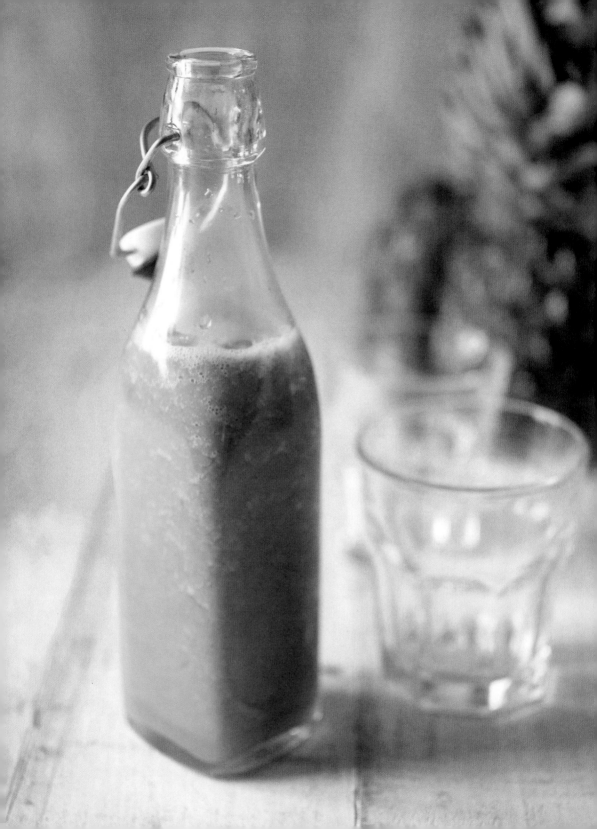

Gingered pineapple revitalizer

A wonderful bright green juice, although the vegetables take a back seat in this naturally sweet tummy-soothing blend. Pineapple not only aids digestion and helps to fight infection, but the enzyme 'bromelain' that it contains may also help to reduce bruising.

1 Add all the ingredients to a blender goblet, secure the lid and blitz until smooth. Pour into a tall glass and serve.

COOK'S TIP – Pineapples vary in size and price, so if yours is bigger or smaller just aim for 200g/7oz/1 cup of prepared pineapple cut into chunks for this juice.

GORGEOUS GINGER – Ginger is regarded as an excellent 'carminative', a substance that promotes the elimination of excessive gas from the digestive system and soothes the intestinal tract. It can also help with travel sickness and morning sickness in pregnancy too. It does have a strong peppery taste so use sparingly; it is always better to add a little extra to a drink after blitzing or juicing if you want to up the strength.

BLEND SERVES 1

¼ medium pineapple, peeled, cored, cut into chunks

1 kiwi fruit, peeled, cut into chunks

5mm/¼in thick slice fresh root ginger, no need to peel, cut into pieces

25g/1oz or 8 sugar snap peas

25g/1oz/1 cup baby spinach leaves

250ml/8fl oz/1 cup water

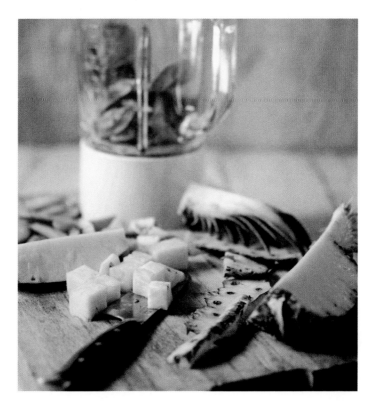

Energy 126kcal/538kJ; Protein 3g; Carbohydrate 28.2g, of which sugars 27.7g; Fat 0.9g, of which saturates 0g; Cholesterol 0mg; Calcium 107mg; Fibre 5.9g; Sodium 42mg.

Index

A
Age Defier 121
almond milk 19, 55, 70, 74, 96, 121
almonds 44, 48, 70, 110, 117
antioxidants 16
  Antioxidant Superfusion 106
apples 26, 51, 52, 65, 77, 87, 106, 124, 127, 128, 131, 132
arugula see rocket
avocados 26, 39, 61, 62, 69, 70, 117

B
bananas 43, 55, 58, 62, 74, 96, 109, 110, 113, 114, 121
baobab 17
  Wake-up Call 51
barley water
  Digestive Soother 109
  First Defence 102
beetroot/beet
  Citrus Beet Blast 65
  Turbo-charged Beet 77
blackberries 58, 69, 121
blender tips 22
blueberries 47, 58, 69, 91
Bone Builder 118
broccoli 26, 36, 40, 43, 87, 92, 99, 106, 114, 118, 132

C
cabbages 27
  Antioxidant Superfusion 106
  Gorgeous Green Pep-up 127
  Red Cabbage and Kale
    Digestive Aid 124
cacao 17
  Cacao and Avocado Smoothie 62
  Cacao Comforter 55
  Cacao Cup 96
carrots 65, 106, 124
cauliflowers 27, 43, 55, 109, 110, 131, 136
celery 27, 40, 80, 87, 88, 124, 128
Chamomile, Pear and Mint
    Pacifier 140
chia seeds 16
  Cacao Cup 96
  Gorgeous Green Pep-up 127
  Kiwi Reviver 83
citrus fruits 26–7
  Citrus Beet Blast 65
  Citrus Burst 52
  Citrus Super-cleanse 135
  First Defence 102
coconut 15, 66
coconut oil 15
coconut milk 15, 36, 62
coconut water 15, 39, 48, 61, 66, 77, 95, 114, 117

courgettes 27, 43, 73, 84, 99, 124, 127, 132
cucumbers 27, 40, 51, 80, 83, 87, 88, 99

D
dairy-free milks 15, 19, 36, 44, 55, 58, 62, 70, 74, 96, 113, 121
detoxing 32
  weekly plan 33
diet 30
  diet plan 30
  staying on track 30
  weekly plan 31
Digestive Soother 109

F
fats 14–15
fennel
  Spring Clean 136
five-a-day 11
flaxseeds 16, 47, 70, 96, 105, 121

G
ginger 36, 87, 92, 102, 109, 132, 143
goji berries 17, 44, 58, 62, 91, 114, 121
Good Morning Shake 48
grapes 27, 48, 51, 61, 69, 88, 109, 127, 136
Green Giant 39
Green Goddess 84
Green Tornado 61

H
Healthy Heart 113
Heartburn Healer 110
hemp 12, 48, 69, 73, 80, 96, 121, 128
herbs 27, 51, 95, 105, 117, 128, 139, 140
Hormone Balance – Men 117
Hormone Balance – Women 114
hydration 17

I
Immune Booster 105
ingredients A-Z 26–29

J
juices 6–9
  juicer tips 24
  making juices 24
  why green juices are good for us 10–11

K
kale 28, 36, 39, 44, 47, 48, 55, 58, 61, 62, 65, 69, 77, 80, 105, 106,

113, 114, 117, 118, 124, 135
kiwi fruit 28, 39, 44, 83, 84, 95, 105, 117, 139, 143

L
lacuma 14
  Minted Melon Crush 95
  Super-green Vitality 80
lettuce 28, 52, 58, 87, 88, 109, 140

M
mangoes
  Totally Tropical 36
melon 84, 91, 92, 95, 139, 140
minerals 15
mint 51, 95, 139, 140

N
nut milks 19, 55, 70, 74, 96, 121
nutrition 12–21

O
oats 13, 44, 58, 113
organic produce 21

P
papaya
  Heartburn Healer 110
  Papaya Passion 66
  Stamina Maximizer 70
parsley
  Immune Booster 105
  Parslied Purifier 128
  Summer Herb Sensation 139
parsnips
  Creamy Apple and Parsnip
    Soother 131
  Red Cabbage and Kale
    Digestive Aid 124
passion fruits
  Hormone Balance – Women 114
  Papaya Passion 66
pea protein
  Cacao Cup 96
  Good morning shake 48
  Green Giant 39
pea shoots 29
  Papaya Passion 66
pears 28, 44, 48, 73, 80, 92, 96, 105, 113, 118, 127, 135, 136, 140
peas, sugar snap
  Gingered Pineapple Revitalizer 143
  Healthy Heart 113
pineapple 36, 40, 77, 83, 99, 143
proteins 12

R
rocket 29
  Summer Salad Bowl 88

Wake-up Call 51

S
sea salad/vegetables 29
  Age Defier 121
  Hormone Balance – Women 114
seeds 16–17, 44, 47, 48, 62, 69, 70, 96, 105, 114, 117, 121
  Ground Seed Mix 47, 62, 70, 105, 114, 117
  pumpkin seeds 48
  sunflower seeds 44, 69
smoothies, making 22
spinach 29, 39, 40, 43, 51, 61, 65, 70, 73, 74, 83, 84, 91, 95, 96, 102, 105, 110, 128, 131, 135, 136, 143
spirulina 16, 40, 113, 132
Stamina Maximizer 70
substitutions 19–20
sugars 13–14
Summer Salad Bowl 88
super-nutrients 16–17
Super-powered Berry Bonanza 58
Swiss Mix 44

T
tea, chamomile
  Chamomile, Pear and Mint
    Pacifier 140
tea, green 16
  Citrus Burst 52
tomatoes
  Hormone Balance – Men 117
Totally Tropical 36

V
vitamins 15
  Vitamin C Supercharge 47

W
Wake-up Call 51
water 17
watercress 29
  Bone Builder 118
  Broccoli and Watercress
    Spritzer 92
watermelon
  Blueberry Booster 91
wheatgrass 17, 29, 44, 124

Y
yogurt 47, 66, 69, 110, 114, 118

Z
Zingy Refresher 40
zucchini see courgettes

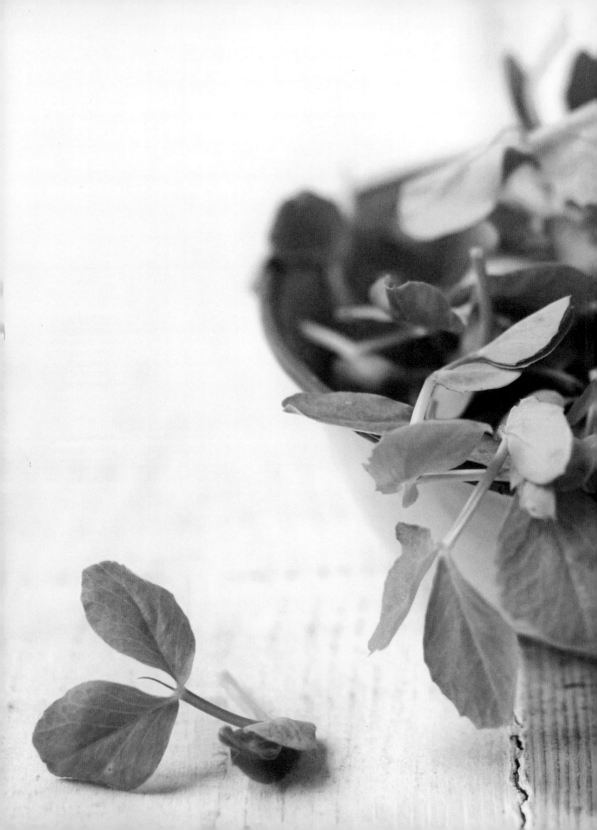